DOCTOR TO PATIENT

LIVING WITH

STIFF PERSON SYNDROME

DOCTOR TO PATIENT

LIVING WITH

STIFF PERSON SYNDROME

DR. TRACY SCOTT

wordeee
where words connect

Nonfiction
Doctor to Patient: Living with Stiff Person Syndrome

ISBN: 978-1-959811-60-2 (Paperback)
ISBN: 978-1-959811-61-9 (e-book)
Library of Congress Control Number: 2022912287

Cover Designer: Christina Panagiotis
Interior Design: Amit Dey
Author Photo: Sarah Bass
Editor: Sarah Bass/AE Williams

Published by Wordeee in the United States New York, New York 2025
Website: www.wordeee.com
X Formerly Twitter: wordeeeupdates
Facebook: facebook.com/wordage/
e-mail: contact@wordeee.com

ADVANCE PRAISE

"*In Doctor to Patient: Living with Stiff Person Syndrome*, Dr. Tracy Scott gives us a unique personal snapshot of what it is like to be diagnosed with Stiff Person Syndrome. His expertise is drawn from years of scientific and clinical experience in neuropsychology. The transforming aspect of this book is Dr. Scott's spiritually artful way of imparting knowledge and developing a plan for coping with this chronic, unpredictable, and lesser-known condition. His navigation of the health care system and his ability to impart hope to fellow humans with Stiff Person Syndrome are invaluable. The duality of his roles as doctor and patient is essential to his message of empowerment and survival."

—Dr. Patricia A. Pimental, President/CEO
Neurobehavioral Medicine Consultants Ltd.
Associate Professor, Behavioral Sciences, Midwestern University
Author, Neuropsychological Aspects of Right Brain Injury

"Living with Stiff Person Syndrome is a daily battle but watching Dr. Scott navigate through it with grace and resilience has been nothing short of inspiring. Despite the constant pain and challenges he faces, his unwavering spirit and determination shine through. One of the most remarkable things about him is how he approaches each day with a sense of humor and empathy, turning even the toughest moments into opportunities for laughter and connection. His ability to find joy in the midst of pain is a true testament to his strength and character.

Through the journey with Stiff Person Syndrome, he has taught us all the power of empathy, laughter, and love in overcoming adversity. He reminds us that even in the darkest of times, there is always room for hope and light. I am grateful to have him in my life, showing me what true courage and resilience look like."

—Joan Mitchell, CRNA, MSHA, BSN, RN

"Dr. Tracy Scott's book, *Doctor to Patient: Living with Stiff Person Syndrome*, offers a deeply personal and informative account of living with a rare and debilitating condition. The text serves both as a memoir and a guide, detailing the challenges faced by those with Stiff-Person Syndrome (SPS) while also providing a broader perspective on chronic and invisible illnesses.

Dr. Scott's narrative is grounded in his personal journey, which adds a layer of authenticity and emotional depth. His candid descriptions of the physical and emotional toll of SPS make the reader empathize with his struggles. Additionally, the manuscript excels in educating the reader about SPS, a condition that many may not be familiar with. The detailed explanations of symptoms, treatments, and the diagnostic process are both informative and accessible, making the book a valuable resource for patients and healthcare providers alike.

As a clinician with extensive experience in neuropsychology and behavioral medicine, Dr. Scott provides a unique perspective that bridges the gap between patient and doctor. His professional insights into the psychological impact of chronic illness add depth to the narrative.

The manuscript emphasizes the importance of empathy and understanding in treating and interacting with individuals with chronic illnesses. Dr. Scott's call for greater compassion and his critique of the medical community's often dismissive attitude toward invisible illnesses are powerful and necessary.

Doctor to Patient: Living with Stiff-Person Syndrome is a valuable contribution to the literature on chronic illness, providing both a personal memoir and a practical guide. Dr. Tracy Scott's manuscript has the potential to be a powerful and influential book. It offers hope, education, and a call for greater empathy and understanding for those living with invisible illnesses."

—*Maria Aparicio, Ph.D.*

"Although Stiff Person Syndrome is a rare disorder, it can significantly affect a patient's quality of life; I sincerely enjoyed reading it. This book should be distributed in markets, public areas, health institutions, schools, and other public areas and social platforms to be accessible to those in need.

I highly appreciated Dr. Scott's amazing job. I found the book very interesting, feasible, and applicable. I believe that it will benefit many professionals and patients, as well as communities in control of chronic diseases and Stiff Person Syndrome."

—*Teklay Kahsay, BSc, Public Health*

"Once I started reading, I couldn't put this book down—as a caregiver for two family members, it spoke to me on a personal level. It's an invaluable resource for anyone dealing with Stiff Person Syndrome or chronic health issues, and it also offers valuable insights for their caregivers and family members.

The coping mechanisms and motivation provided in this book will help me live a better life while taking care of my loved ones with chronic illnesses. One of my favorite part of the book was learning about the remedies to relieve symptoms—it brought me joy and hope. Dr. Scott's explanation of empathy vs. compassion was eye-opening, as was your determination to make positive changes in your life to manage Stiff Person Syndrome. It's truly inspiring and can encourage readers to do the same. The section on how society is ill-equipped to handle those with invisible chronic illnesses was enlightening and will help me interact more effectively with my family members in need of care.

As a caregiver, I know the weight of responsibility and sacrifice that comes with the role, but this book has given me the motivation to not only provide better care but also take charge of my health and advocate for myself when faced with a chronic illness."

—Pamela Gee Hall, Caregiver

"This book provides a deeply personal and insightful account of Dr. Scott's journey living with Stiff Person Syndrome (SPS). After going undiagnosed for more than a decade, Dr. Scott talks about his struggle with identifying his source of pain. He excels in describing non-traditional treatments, offering a valuable perspective on alternative approaches to managing this rare condition. It beautifully underscores the profound connection between mind, body, and spirit, emphasizing its critical role in holistic healing. Additionally, the exploration of living with an invisible illness sheds light on the often-overlooked aspects of empathy and understanding of those living with SPS, making this a compelling and enlightening read for all."

—Sheryl A Neverson, Ph.D., LCSW-C, LICSW
CEO, Transitions Therapeutic Services

DISCLOSURE AND LEGAL DISCLAIMER

This book provides guidance for living with Stiff Person Syndrome and is not intended as a substitute for the medical or psychological advice of physicians, psychologists, and/or other healthcare professionals. The reader should consult their healthcare team in matters relating to his/her/their health and particularly concerning any symptoms that may require diagnosis or medical attention. Healthcare decisions should be made collaboratively between you and your healthcare providers.

This book contains links to external websites, references, or resources maintained by third parties. These links and references are provided for convenience and do not signify endorsement or responsibility for the content, accuracy, or availability of these external resources. Dr. Scott and the Publisher shall not be held liable for any damages or loss arising from the use of such external links.

Dr. Scott has tried to recreate events, locales, and conversations from his memories of them. To maintain their anonymity in some instances he has changed the names of individuals and places, some identifying characteristics and details such as physical properties, occupations, and places of residence. Dr. Scott and the Publisher hold no liability for decisions made based on this book.

DEDICATION

In memory of my parents, Linette and Susie Scott,
whose examples of living with chronic health issues
taught me many invaluable lessons.

FOREWORD

Taking it from a very esoteric academic, it was a dynamic privilege and honor to review this manuscript. It offers a billion dollars' worth of therapy to many readers, especially all with minimal finances to afford the best medical treatments! Dr. Scott has distilled, with great empathy and tact, decades of professional experience as an educator and healthcare provider into a tractable book for those with Stiff Person Syndrome and similar illnesses.

The book contains a plethora of wisdom, practical insights, and pertinent case studies or realistic examples from the career of a dedicated healer who now experiences a debilitating disease with helpful optimism and protracted hope. The contents of this treatise were not rushed, allowing the readers to be converted to its therapy—a wealth of pertinent expertise.

The book begins with helpful disclaimers about its purposes and limitations. Thereafter, it is smooth, creative, and engaging with clarity as well as superb writing. Dr. Scott is an articulate medical professional, who shares his motivations, experiences, and struggles with adroit intentionality! He discloses his misgivings, anxieties, traumas, loneliness, isolation, vulnerabilities, and limitations in battling Stiff Person Syndrome. He invites the reader into his personal and professional life, a rare occurrence for medical professionals.

The medical and clinical expertise he provides is priceless, along with his documentation of helpful resources to guide readers to additional information about chronic illnesses. Moreover, he delivers methods for overcoming the insufficiencies of the healthcare system. His elaborations about and interactions with Annika and Betty are stunning as well as inspirational. The comments about the social or communal aspects of healing bring tears, inviting the readers to a symphony of empathy. Yet, Dr. Scott integrates the clinical and medical research well throughout the manuscript with sustained, appropriate critique where needed!

Pertinent expertise exudes from this book, regarding topics such as empathy, compassion, avoidance, detachment, social learning theory, caring, sensitivity, and similar phenomena. His comments about cannabis are mandatory, and therapeutic with relevant guidelines and sources. I was convicted regarding his insights about gratitude, laughter, meditation, diet, sex, and pharmacology. Priceless expertise was interwoven with practicable projects, sustainable for all!

Our society and world need authentic love, compassion, and empathy. These valuable, incalculable commodities energize health, especially for anyone with Stiff Person Syndrome and chronic illness. Dr. Scott has written a monumental book that captures their essence.

—Dr. Henry Allen, Ph.D., Sociology

PREFACE

Beloved and Almighty Creator,

I want to express my gratitude for allowing me to find solace in You. Your strength and power are beyond measure, and I am grateful for your constant presence in my life.

Thanks to your guidance, I have transformed into a person of integrity who values honesty and treats others fairly. Deceitful acts hold no place in my life: instead, I despise lies and bribes. My inner strength allows me to resist the temptation of corruption, jealousy, and envy. When faced with adversity, I do not lose my temper or harbor resentment towards others. Instead, I approach each challenge with a level head and a sense of responsibility.

However, this morning when I looked in the mirror, I realized that everything I had thought was real was just a dream.

On Thursday, December 8, 2022, a year after canceling her concert residency in Las Vegas, news of the six-time Grammy Award-winner's incurable condition spread worldwide. The famous 54-year-old singer's cancelation of her tour was due to a rare neurological disorder that affected her singing and movement abilities called Stiff Person Syndrome. Doctors have confirmed it as the cause of her persistent muscle spasms, greatly impacting her daily life and stage performances.[1] In 2024 she detailed her health battle in a documentary, *I AM Celine Dion*. When Celine Dion first publicized her diagnosis, the Stiff Person Syndrome community could relate to her words. I have been a part of this group since 2017, and like other members, I understood exactly what she meant.

As Celine Dion's announcement spread through the Stiff Person Syndrome community, I couldn't help but think of my journey with the chronic illness. Like Celine, I had struggled to complete even the simplest of tasks some days, my body wracked with spasms and pain. But unlike Celine, as a healthcare professional, the irony of the situation was not lost on me. I had spent my career helping others navigate the complex landscape of chronic illness. Yet, despite being a doctor, I now found myself a patient diagnosed with SPS and I knew all too well the struggles she would be facing and the difficulties of performing on stage with stiff muscles and spasms.

I wanted to write a book that would be helpful for those suffering from Stiff Person Syndrome and those who care about them—such as spouses, relatives, and friends. Chronic health problems like this one have a wide-reaching effect on an individual's life and those around them. However, to make the best impact on those with SPS, it is essential to understand how this condition influences every aspect of their life.

The focus of the work is to be a resource for understanding the medical and psychological implications of having SPS. It delves into how it affects an individual's mental and social well-being and activities of daily life. It's meant to serve as a tool rather than a memoir.

Writing this book was a toilsome and arduous process that occurred in various places. I wrote while lying in bed, riding in the car, taking short walks, watching movies, and tapping away on my cell phone. I wrote whenever I could. Notes were all over the office floor, taped to the wall, and scattered across my desk. On some days, I ended up overworking myself, and I would have to take a break for several days or even weeks.

Then, at times, the spasms would be so severe that I was unable to organize my thoughts. These stretches made it impossible for me to work on it, and weeks would pass between attempts. On occasions, the physical pain of the spasms weighed so heavily on me that, during my toughest moments, I found myself contemplating giving up on the project entirely, feeling incapable of ever finishing it. But I refused to give up. I knew that the information was important. Nonetheless, one day, it was done. The manuscript was complete, and all that was left was to send it to the publisher and make it available for others to read.

While the book was crafted to be beneficial for individuals with Stiff Person Syndrome, it is also for the people in their lives who are there to support them—loved ones, partners, and associates alike. I am especially hoping that doctors, therapists, and other healthcare professionals will find value in reading the book; people struggling with chronic health conditions rely heavily upon expert guidance. Thus, some sections of the book are purposely opined in a clinical tone. However, people who lack a medical or psychology background but are working with individuals with chronic illness, perhaps as caregivers, will also gain valuable information from its content. It also offers an introduction to medical and psychology terms and concepts, making it a great supplementary reader for students.

Each chapter also includes a Learning and Discussion Section, allowing readers to bolster their comprehension of key topics and apply the book's knowledge to their personal lives, fostering self-assurance in overcoming struggles. Because SPS is so new and mysterious, I have included a lot of references for people who seek to learn more than can be written in this book.

My written voice in this book comes from both my clinical perspective and also my experience as a patient. I am neither one of these exclusively, but perhaps, rather, something deeper.

Tracy Scott

TABLE OF CONTENT

CHAPTER ONE

MYSTERY ILLNESS

It was around 2004 when I began to have little spasms. They were small at first and would crop up out of nowhere in different isolated parts of my body. They were annoying, but I initially thought nothing of it because they would quickly resolve themselves. I thought, "Maybe I'm just having cramps." The problem was, I wasn't doing any strenuous physical activity. I wasn't playing sports, and having been a former athlete, I knew what brought on cramps as a part of my training. These weren't anything like that, as they seemed to be triggered by anything I was doing.

Early on, the spasms would come on, then go away on their own. I was able to ignore them because they were small. With time, though, they began to occur more frequently and were slowly increasing in intensity. I also began to experience whole-body stiffness around this time, particularly when the ambient temperature dropped to 50 degrees Fahrenheit (10 degrees Celsius) or when I was cold. The stiffness would be so significant that I felt like a 2x4 plank attempting to bend after being removed from the freezer. At times, I resembled the Tin Man featured in *The Wizard of Oz*.[1] I was barely able to move. And while the stiffness is problematic, the spasms are debilitating.

This started me on a search to try to understand what was going on in my body. I considered the possibility that it was medication-related since many medications can produce spasms. Or, perhaps I was somehow vitamin-deficient, or lacking in enzymes. Maybe something was off in my blood chemistry. If there were things I could adjust or add to my diet to improve it, I was committed to doing it. I therefore focused my attention on my nutrition. The spasms, however, persisted.

In an attempt to relax my muscles, I began getting into the hot shower. This, in addition to hot baths, became my new method of making the spasms dissipate. Despite all this, the gradual escalation continued, and it was alarming. "Okay, maybe I'm doing too much," I said to myself. "My body is clearly exhausted and overworked. I need rest."

I made it a point to be intentional about taking it easy. Then, one day, while I was in the shower, the spasms came on. It was then that I began to wonder if I was dealing with a more serious medical issue. I went to my doctor and explained what I was experiencing. He ran some tests. When the tests came back my bloodwork was pristine. Everything was normal! That's when I became really concerned because while there appeared to be nothing wrong, the spasms were getting progressively worse.

My doctor didn't have a diagnosis for me. He recommended that I visit a specialist at a pain clinic. The day I went to the pain clinic for intervention and treatment, I was in the middle of explaining my symptoms to the doctor when all of a sudden, spasms erupted all over my body. It scared the doctor. He and the medical staff had never seen anything like it. They began injecting me with what is called Trigger Point Injections (TPI, saline, and corticosteroid in an attempt to calm my physical response down. I had never experienced anything so drastic in my entire life. And yet, despite more tests, the doctor couldn't tell me what was wrong.

The specialists, too, were confounded. All they could do was try and help me manage the excruciating pain that accompanied the episodes. TPI worked, momentarily. But by the time I returned home, the spasms were again starting to erupt.

Since the hot showers, baths, sauna, and all the other natural methods I'd taken to alleviate the spasms stopped working, the pain specialist prescribed Baclofen. Baclofen is a muscle relaxant and antispastic. It's effective for the alleviation of signs and symptoms of spasticity resulting from multiple sclerosis, flexor spasms, and muscular rigidity.[2] Baclofen helped, until the spasms began to break through the Baclofen, rendering it ineffective.

Around 2015, I switched primary care doctors and was referred to another pain specialist. This doctor started me on a series of new treatments, but not only were they ineffective, but every time they'd do an intervention, the spasms seemed to worsen.

One afternoon, the doctor, who was aware of my healthcare background, sat me down. "Dr. Scott, look," he said. "I'd like to talk to you about something. Have you ever heard of a disease called Stiff Person Syndrome?"

"Stiff Person Syndrome?" I repeated. "No, I haven't."

"I would like for you to go home and look it up. Then, you and I need to talk," he said.

I left his office, went down to the parking lot, and sat in the car. I decided to look up Stiff Person Syndrome right then and there. When I saw the presentation of the syndrome and read up on its description and symptoms, I was looking at myself. Up to this point, the medical professionals had thought that perhaps it was fibromyalgia or some other chronic arthritic condition

I had since I also suffered from arthritis. But witnessing video testimonials and seeing the nature of the spasms individuals with Stiff Person Syndrome were experiencing—specifically their onset, intensity, and the pain that accompanied them—I knew right away that I had my answer. "My God!" I said aloud. "This is exactly what it is!" After nearly a decade and a half of seeing specialists producing inconclusive and inaccurate diagnoses, I finally had my answer.

The question now was, what to do about it?

Classification of Terms

Illness, syndrome, and disease are three terms that are often used interchangeably, but they have different meanings. Distinguishing between the three can be complicated, convoluted, and confusing, especially for the general population. In reality, an illness is your understanding of how it feels to feel in poor health or have a feeling of discomfort or pain, which may or may not be associated with a specific disease or medical condition. However, a syndrome is a recognizable composite of symptoms and physical findings that indicate a particular condition for which an exact cause is not necessarily understood. But once medical science pinpoints a cause, or the pathology of the condition, it may then be referred to as a disease.[3]

Additionally, the use of the term chronic disease refers to long lasting conditions that usually can be controlled but not cured and the symptoms can vary between periods of exacerbation and remission. While on the other hand, chronic illness signifies your understanding or personal experience of living with a disease. More specifically, to what degree do your symptoms affect your personal, social, work, and financial quality of life?[4]

So, What is SPS?

Stiff-Person Syndrome (SPS) falls into the classification of chronic disease. It is a syndrome because it presents with symptoms with no cause of origin and is believed to be a neurological condition caused by an autoimmune disease that attacks the central nervous system that controls muscle movement. Apart from muscle stiffness, painful spasms, depression, and anxiety, it can also make people who are affected sensitive to noise, touch, movements such as twisting, bending, or turning, and emotional distress, which can also trigger spasm attacks.

The spasms can start in the feet, legs, and abdomen before moving to other body parts, including the neck, arms, or upper trunk. My spasms often start in my legs, feet, arms, or hands before engulfing several areas simultaneously. The spasms are excruciating and can be unbearable. My legs are embedded with scar tissue from the numerous spasms.

SPS generally develops in the early mid-life ages between 40-50, but it is not limited to this developmental stage. There is no known cure for SPS. While there is no known cure, there is hope that a new medication that at the time of this writing is being used to treat people with a refractory manifestation, one of the variants of Stiff-Person Syndrome, will soon be available to the public. More testing needs to be done.[5]

Diagnosis as Trauma

As a retired clinician who spent a large portion of his career working in the hospital, I am accustomed to the clinical side of the diagnostic process. This included assessing a patient's condition based on the underlying psychological, biopsychological, and even spiritual factors present, and assisting them in addressing those things. We would then use those conclusions to determine the level of care needed, develop care and crisis management plans, and help patients understand the implications of their prognosis. This degree of intimacy required the establishment of trust between the doctor and the patient.

Developing a trusting relationship between doctor and patient is a magical yet humbling experience. It requires an authenticity that cannot be falsified. That being said, each and every doctor-patient encounter provides opportunities for making discoveries, confronting challenges, and providing encouragement. I always approached the care of my patients with the intent to help them through the emotional turmoil that often accompanies a traumatic diagnosis.

In 2017, I was a patient in a similar situation, needing the support of my doctor. After hearing the words "Stiff Person Syndrome" for the first time, I was relieved because I finally had something concrete. Now that I could name my diagnosis, I was committed to learning all I could about this rare disease. But, I underestimated the traumatic effect the identification of my disease would have on me. While having all the information I could ingest about SPS was important, it was also a profoundly upsetting realization. I had a medical condition that had no cure.

Furthermore, when I returned to my pain specialist's office the week following his suggested diagnosis, I was now officially in the role of the patient. Sitting in the waiting room, I was familiar with the steps that would ensue, because I had walked hundreds of patients through them. Naturally, I assumed that my professional understanding of disease processes, and the mental preparedness I had obtained through my experience that was now required for my journey, would put me at a psychological advantage. Yet sitting there, waiting to see my doctor, and observing other patients arrive for their appointments, I felt my anxiety begin to surface.

The more I processed the presumed diagnosis of SPS, for which there were few known treatment options and no available cure, the more concerns and questions about my future flooded my mind. What did I stand to lose? What would happen to my mobility and cognition? Would my family be okay if I declined? How long could I live in a debilitated state? What medical equipment would I need? Is my home wheelchair accessible?

"This can't be happening to me," I thought. "Why is this happening to me?" I was suddenly overwhelmed by the sense that there was a ticking bomb inside of me.

Throughout my professional career, I've lost count of how many times I've been the deliverer of tough, life-changing news. I knew the right words to say and had extensive training in how to provide comfort. Now, I was on the receiving end of traumatic news, and it was a different, unfamiliar, and unwelcome experience.

As a clinician, I was accustomed to being in control of the healthcare environment. This was also true of my role as a professor. When I became a patient, however, I was forced to relinquish all perceived authority over the situation, because I was no longer the person with the answers.

Even though I was fortunate to have a compassionate doctor who was clear and thorough in his confirmation and explanation of my diagnosis, it was still a lonely, traumatic experience. Over the next few weeks, I was overwhelmed by a flood of emotions. Despite the fact my wife and children were supportive, I felt very isolated and alone. There were moments when I would feel somewhat "normal;" when I was temporarily distracted at the moment teasing my wife, watching a funny movie, or discussing life issues with my daughters. In those moments, which I cherished, I could temporarily forget about the journey I was now on. But when the world went quiet and I was left with my own thoughts, I was forced to confront the chaotic universe of my altered life; a universe in which I was looking at a future full of concern, trepidation, and uncertainty. Now that I was a patient, I was overcome with worry and a feeling of powerlessness. I was also afraid, as I realized that my experience and knowledge couldn't protect me from the terror of my reality.

As I grew in awareness of my new limitations, vulnerabilities, and the resulting loss of self-esteem, I was concerned that I was at risk of depression. This was common among people diagnosed with a serious, life-changing chronic illness or disease. After a diagnosis of a serious illness, feelings of sadness and despair are normal."[6]

One day while I was driving and listening to worship music, I suddenly began to cry. I was overwhelmed by my anxiety at having SPS, my fears of being disabled, and feelings of guilt that I somehow brought this on myself and was the person responsible for allowing the disease to propagate in my body. I phoned my wife for support, but as the anxiety increased, I realized that I was, for the first time in my life, experiencing a panic attack.

In that moment of emotional and psychological crisis, I was neither Dr. nor Professor Scott, but simply human in my shortcomings, frailties, sorrow, and pain. I was, however, well aware of the fact that for any individual, couple, or family, one of the best ways to address, fix, deal with, or confront these critical encounters is to seek counseling. When the conversation with my wife ended, I immediately contacted my primary care doctor for an appointment. Providentially, an opening was available that day, so I headed to his office.

My doctor, thankfully, understood the emotional impact of receiving a chronic illness diagnosis and spoke with me in a sensitive, honest, and candid manner. Regrettably, for many people who suffer from chronic illnesses, one of their most challenging tasks is finding a doctor who understands the mental health impact of the disease and, in light of that, provides a much-needed support and treatment plan. This may not, however, always be the case. Although medical doctors may possess the necessary tools and knowledge to tend to the physical aspects of treatment, it is essential for them to also address the intricate complexities of a patient's mental, emotional, and cultural well-being. This holistic approach to healthcare is crucial in providing comprehensive and effective care.[7] Unfortunately, my anxiety continued during the visit, so he prescribed medication for generalized anxiety.

Doctor to Patient

I entered the field of psychology because, as a kid growing up in the inner city of Chicago, I was determined to commit my life to helping others. It was a mission-driven intent fueled by dedication and determination to care for others when they need it most.

I was an energetic professional with a doctorate in clinical psychology, specializing in clinical neuropsychology. In the late '80s and early '90s, I completed an externship, internship, and two-year postdoctoral fellowship in clinical psychology and clinical neuropsychology. My patient load primarily consisted of people with traumatic brain and spinal cord injuries from the inner city of Chicago. Furthermore, while working at a top pharmaceutical company, I gained advanced knowledge in neuroscience and psychopharmacology. Additionally, I had clinical training in African, Black, and Christian psychology and was an ordained clergy. For many years, I was the host of two online radio programs and the featured guest of a terrestrial radio program that aired in Milwaukee, Wisconsin, and Eudora, Arkansas.

In 2009, I was on the faculty of a major university teaching psychology courses. I had a long history of faculty appointments dating back to 1992 and received recognition as a clinician and professor. I had worked hard to earn my degrees and experiences. I was proud of what I did every day and enjoyed it. However, I understood that my training and career path were unique. I was among the few with highly specialized education and training in clinical psychology, clinical neuropsychology, psychopharmacology, and clinical spiritual counseling. I was active in my community, providing seminars and workshops on various topics to help promote good emotional health. In addition, I was a husband and a father.

Earning a doctorate is not easy; it takes exceptional hard work and perseverance. Yet, while working hard to develop diverse and expert knowledge, we must remain human. I was right there—in the corridor for success, persisting in fulfilling my dreams. Now in its place, I inadvertently entered into the treacherous world of chronic illness —and my horror, discovered there was no cure or way out.

Chronic Illness

While numerous people are diagnosed with a disease, disorder, or injury every day, many will be diagnosed with a condition that has a short duration, requiring brief therapy or treatment. Conversely, six in ten Americans will go on to live with at least one chronic disease that is long lasting and incurable.[8] Sometimes chronic illness can be treated and managed, with some people able to work and live without becoming extremely sick and incapacitated. Others, however, who are living with a chronic illness may find it difficult to participate in everyday activities, especially if the condition is progressive and worsens with time. And mind you SPS affects one to two people in a million!

It's important to understand that some people with chronic illnesses face invisible obstacles and may look completely healthy on the outside. Their symptoms and the severity of them are not necessarily conspicuous, a fact that can lead to a lack of understanding and support from their co-workers, treatment team, family members, and friends.[9] Chronic diseases are the leading causes of death and disability in America[10] and are the main contributors to both fatalities and disabilities. They are also the most widespread, expensive, and leading cause of death compared to all other health conditions, claiming the lives of seven out of every ten individuals impacted.[11]

It is clear from medical research that people living with chronic illnesses must adapt to the constant and unpredictable changes in their condition. Many experience anxiety and worry about their illness returning or worsening. Individuals who have survived cancer often describe this feeling as a constant fear, similar to the threat of the sword of Damocles hanging over them for the rest of their lives.[12] I, however, wasn't worried about cancer; I was concerned about the probability and projected rate of my deterioration from Stiff Person Syndrome.

Hindsight

Looking back, I guess it's easy to get into a plunging state of mind and withdraw when you receive this type of information. You can, without effort, be consumed with negativity. I was scared and began to realize that my experience and knowledge couldn't protect me from what was happening. This situation was no dream.

I have practiced self-care throughout my professional career. While teaching graduate psychology students, I stress the importance of caring for oneself. And by that, I mean to take care of one's emotional, physical, and spiritual needs so one can grow healthy in their personal and professional development. Although there is autonomy, independence, and variability in how self-care occurs, I routinely provide these suggestions: develop three to five people with whom you can share your innermost thoughts; seek supervision; have more than one hobby; find time to laugh; consistently exercise; eat a proper diet; find time for worship; and seek medical and psychological help if needed. I was aware of the importance of seeking help because we were required to (personally) undergo individual and group counseling during my doctorate program as a part of our maturation as clinicians.

Additionally, while the suggestions were a part of my foundation, they were insufficient to help me deal with the emotions I was experiencing. Unlike the counseling I experienced as a graduate student, I was confronted with being a forever patient this time. I had used up all my skills, suggestions, self-talk, and cognitive restructuring techniques, and I was getting worse. I needed someone there to ensure I did not fall through the cracks.

Knowing I had an advocate in my doctor, and having walked this journey with him, I trusted him. I felt so reassured. On my way home from his office, my anxiety subsided and never returned. I was therefore able to discontinue the anxiety medication.

Aesop was correct, as usual. A person with a severe malady should be very cautious about treating himself because he who treats himself has a fool for a patient.[13] Even though I have deep experience in understanding how the brain and the mind function when injured or met with adversities, I am not the best person to recognize and treat my faulty thinking.

The next day, I contacted one of my mentors, and she gladly offered to help. It was time to stop being the doctor and transform into the patient. I was now trying to understand my new normal. Today I know you don't get a test run at learning how to move from doctor to becoming a patient; you learn as you go. So, the following week, the counseling sessions began.

LEARNING AND DISCUSSION: SUGGESTIONS FOR SELECTING A "GOOD DOCTOR?"

In your lifetime, there will be moments when you must make important decisions about your health. During this time of decision-making, many questions are swirling in your head. You might feel perplexed, confused, overwhelmed, or bewildered as you try to answer questions such as: How do you determine the best course of action? What resources do you rely on, and are they trustworthy? Will you have the necessary knowledge when you need it most? To answer these questions, you might seek advice from family or friends, read books and magazines, or browse websites for information. However, you cannot know if they are objective or if the information you've gathered is factual. At this moment, having a compatible, competent, and dedicated doctor who demonstrates honesty, compassion, empathy, and respect can be priceless. The collaboration between you, an informed patient, and a dedicated doctor can greatly improve, minimize, or alleviate various health concerns. Nevertheless, finding a doctor with these qualities can be time-consuming and difficult. In spite of this, as the leader of your healthcare journey, you have the final decision and must decide who will provide you with the care you deserve.

Here are five behaviors and or qualities that, in my opinion, make a "good doctor." I hope this information aids you in your journey through the healthcare system as you search for a suitable doctor who meets your specific needs.

- **A good doctor is someone who is a true, passionate ally**

An ardent, supportive healthcare provider is one who is deeply involved with their patients, aware of how to guide them through difficult times, and determined to provide the necessary resources for healing.

Imagine this scenario: you've been experiencing persistent swelling and pain in your abdomen area, and despite trying over-the-counter remedies, it won't go away. In this case, scheduling an appointment with your primary care physician is imperative. While you may not be aware of the potential dangers of your symptoms, your doctor will have a better understanding and can guide you toward the most appropriate specialist or facility. In this situation, they may refer you to a renowned physician specializing in diagnosing and treating the factors that caused the swelling and pain. However, a truly exceptional doctor goes above and beyond simply diagnosing and prescribing treatments. They will also serve as your advocate within the healthcare system, working tirelessly to ensure you receive the best care and treatment possible. They can also expertly facilitate communication between different teams of providers, bridging any gaps that may exist and ensuring seamless care coordination for your overall well-being.

- **A good doctor is someone who listens to your opinions and concerns**

A "good doctor" will make every effort to actively and fully listen to your thoughts and concerns without interrupting. Their body language and positioning convey openness and receptiveness, fostering a solid doctor-patient relationship built on trust and satisfaction. They treat patients respectfully and encourage them to speak up and voice any concerns about their treatment options. They have a high regard for the patient's input and ensure they have an equal role in decision-making. Through open communication, "good doctors" provide patients with the necessary information to make the best decisions.

- **A good doctor is well-informed**

Physicians are some of the most knowledgeable people in their area of focus. However, everyone, including doctors and health care providers, are not immune to common reasoning errors like relying too heavily on habits and shortcuts in perception or being overly confident in their abilities. Conversely, "good doctors" demonstrate exceptional knowledge and wisdom by understanding when they encounter a situation that exceeds their expertise and abilities. They also constantly expand their knowledge by staying updated with the latest information and are always eager to pass on their wisdom and skills to educate those around them.

A good doctor is accessible

A welcome surprise about the healthcare service in some smaller countries with less economic wealth, like Panama, Costa Rica, and Cuba, is that doctors normally take the time to sit down and talk to you. You actually feel like you are, in fact, a patient and not a number or insurance claim. You don't feel as though you are there to generate an income stream or to pay the office expenditures. Witnessing a doctor typing on the computer during an office visit and rushing out of the room to get to their next appointment are not a common occurrence. In addition to discussing the reason for your appointment, doctors, take the time to discuss your lifestyle, relationships, or anything that may be causing you stress.

Disturbingly, the medical system in the United States, the pursuit of monetary gain supersedes patient care. Doctors are often bogged down by paperwork, regulations, and excessive caseloads. Most doctors are given a mere fifteen minutes for each routine office visit, and even then, they are constantly interrupted and reminded to move on to the next patient.

This pressure to increase productivity at the cost of quality time with patients leads to difficulty scheduling appointments and long wait times for callbacks. Moreover, still when one does secure an appointment, the waiting room experience seems to last longer than your actual time with the doctor.

On the other hand, a "good doctor" will have a protocol in place for you to reach out regarding any medical concerns, appointments, prescription requests, or questions about test results, even if they cannot be reached right away. They will strive to ensure that either they or one of their colleagues in the practice can respond to you promptly through various means such as phone calls, email portals, text messages, or online telehealth platforms within an appropriate time. Plus, if by chance the doctor is not immediately available at the time of the scheduled appointment, there is no need to worry because a "good doctor" will prioritize your care and give you the attention you deserve once the appointment begins.

- **A good doctor is culturally responsive**

Patients of all ages, races, and backgrounds fill the waiting room, each with their own set of beliefs, struggles, and cultures. "Good doctors" understand and embrace the importance of taking the time to familiarize themselves with different cultures and appreciate how diverse patient backgrounds can significantly enhance a doctor's ability to empathize and connect with their patients.

"Good doctors" strive to listen to and comprehend a patient's story because they know it is crucial to making patients feel understood and validated. Even if they can't personally relate to their patient's experiences, "good doctors" recognize that cultural factors significantly influence how a patient perceives their health situation. Therefore, they are aware of differing world views and examine their own biases, values, and motives while avoiding and rejecting the myth of color blindness. "Good doctors" practice culturally sensitive healthcare by establishing trust and respect and acknowledging culture's impact on a person's beliefs, values, customs, and overall lifestyle.

Think Carefully and Respond to the Following Statements:

How important is it to you that your doctor is competent and compatible with your specific needs? Why?

What other actions and characteristics do you think are necessary for a doctor to exhibit to be considered a "good doctor"?

What questions do you believe are essential to ask a doctor to determine if they are the right fit for your needs?

CHAPTER TWO

THE IMPACT OF LIVING WITH AN INVISIBLE ILLNESS

Stiff Person Syndrome (SPS) also known as Moersch-Woltman Syndrome is hidden from the naked eye. It's a chronic and invisible disease, and no one can discern it unless spasms and/or severe stiffness are present. There are no cosmetic changes by which your body is enhanced, reshaped, or toned. It does not involve the need for a facelift or a tummy tuck. As an SPS patient, I have not lost hair from chemotherapy. I don't have tremors and my speech is fluent. I have no malformations or lesions on the skin, and facial drooping is not one of the symptoms. I don't have visible muscle wasting or the need for a feeding tube. I don't need a back brace, fracture boot, wheelchair, or neck support. Therefore, individuals who see me at the gym, movie theater, store, church, at an event, walking along the beach, or at a sit-down for a conversation in their home would never assume that I have SPS, a chronic illness. By looking at me, you would not realize or understand my daily conflict because the disease is unnoticeable to others.

I don't look feeble, or brittle, or like I'm in poor health, despite experiencing agonizing and unbearable spasms and chronic pain. On the contrary, I am often told that I look good;

about twenty years younger than my age. However, looking good is not a 1:1 relationship to feeling good. I don't look sick, but I am. There are moments when the spasms are so tormenting, that it seems as though my bones are breaking, and without the help of the medication, there would be no relief.

What is an Invisible Illness?

"Invisible" chronic illness (ICI) is defined as an illness that shares the common traits of chronic conditions, but also has the unique quality of being imperceptible, unobservable, and like an invisible cloak, it cloaks its captives in a shroud of secrecy and isolation. Its symptoms are only visible to the one who suffers from it.[1] Invisible conditions are not always well understood by loved ones and are often discounted by family and friends.[2] Because the symptoms of SPS are not always observable, it's usually easier for a loved one to conclude that the signs are fabricated, bogus, or made up. After all, seeing is believing, right? Those without a hidden malady often don't understand how terrifying the disease can be. Illnesses such as cystic fibrosis, pulmonary hypertension, cancer, and lupus, can be life-threatening for some invisible disease sufferers.

This lack of understanding about ICI can lead to feelings of depression, frustration, disappointment, and anger. In fact, encouragement may not come at all, nor help from anyone. The realization that the never-ending support needed to endure the chronic disease may never materialize results in many fractured or terminated relationships.

Sometimes, the lack of understanding can seem overwhelming and, frankly, insuperable. Living in constant pain and with the consequences of a lack of comprehension and support from family and friends can encourage one to isolate and feel helpless. It can create obstacles that will thwart a person's efforts to find joy in life. The outcome gets especially heartrending if a person finds themselves in a relationship with someone—perhaps with a friend or family member—who is unable to put themselves in that person's shoes. My first experience with the sequela of a hidden disease occurred during graduate school while completing my externship in clinical psychology.

As a central part of the Doctor of Psychology in Clinical Psychology program, each student is expected to acquire a broad range of supervised clinical experiences and troubleshoot problems in different settings with various assessment and therapeutic approaches in an increasingly complex and intensive manner. Externs are exposed to diverse roles, populations, settings, and various types of interventions. They are expected to learn to make theory-practice links and apply the knowledge learned in academic teaching. In addition to direct patient care, psychology externs participate in research projects and apply their skills within the clinical setting and in community agencies affiliated with hospitals and clinics. Externs often work in consultation and collaboration with staff from other disciplines. They are an integrated multidisciplinary team member, and they collaborate with clinical team members to provide services and receive direct and ongoing supervision from staff psychologists.

My externship involved a patient named Annika. The experience was life-changing for me. Through clinical supervision and working with Annika, I learned that seeing is not always believing and that sight is limited in understanding reality. Thirty-plus years later, I remember her story as if it occurred yesterday.

Annika's Story

Annika was a 35-year-old, married white female. She was an attractive young woman with natural blonde hair and hazel eyes. Annika appeared to have the physical features that would rival a professional model. She presented in a frank, open, engaging manner, yet she looked distressed and was close to tears when she walked into my office.

When I asked Annika to tell me in her own words what had brought her in to see me, she replied she was having marital difficulties. She reported that her marriage was floundering and on the verge of collapse after her multiple sclerosis and breast cancer diagnoses. Annika reported that her husband stated, "Look at you. There's nothing wrong with you," and strongly encouraged her to find a job and get to work.

"He insists that I work, and suggests I am faking being sick despite having had a double mastectomy and being on medication for multiple sclerosis. He forces me to have sex and attend social events with him. And, if I don't comply, he gets angry. My husband is resentful and emotionally absent. Without the support of my twin sister, who also suffers from multiple sclerosis and breast cancer, I would be alone to deal with the challenges of treatment and recovery," she explained. In tears, she told me that her husband blaming her and being emotionally absent were painful to deal with, but not as painful as accusing her of being deceptive and having bogus diseases. Physically shaking, she said, "After a long wait, I summoned the courage to seek help."

Annika was having trouble sleeping and would often wake up with nightmares. And, along with the chronic health issues of multiple sclerosis, breast cancer, and marital difficulties, she was now depressed. But, physically and aesthetically, there was no way to conclude that Annika suffered from two potentially life-threatening illnesses. Her illness was unseen.

While a treatment plan for Annika's physical and mental health problems was developed, there was no treatment plan for Annika's most challenging issue: her good looks. I suspect she will gather wisdom along the painful journey of looking beautiful to the outside world yet living with a hidden illness. Her beauty was now a curse.

The Difficulty of Empathy

The absence of empathy, compassion, and understanding is not limited to loved ones; it includes medical professionals. Throughout their careers, doctors are pigeonholed to fix, treat, and diagnose people's illnesses. But when individuals present who don't look sick, and they cannot immediately diagnose a disease, medical professionals may quickly dismiss the patient's story. If I can't see or analyze it, it doesn't exist, and I cannot treat it. Unfortunately, this is an acceptable conclusion in the field of medicine. I am very fortunate that that is not my story. However, regarding family, friends, acquaintances, strangers, and the general public, the misconceptions, and pressures to prove that you are ill are very real.

The comments listed below are often heard and identified within the ICI community. And although they are conceivably well-intended, they diminish the gravity of SPS. Moreover, these comments are harmful, primarily when produced within repeated social interactions. They quickly become an incentive for intensification in questioning whether people really care:

- "Brother, you look good. You don't look sick at all."
- "Well, it could be worse. But at least you don't have cancer and haven't lost your mind."

- "You need to see my chiropractor and become a vegan."
- "It would help if you lost weight."
- "Whatever you have, you are dealing with it well."
- "You should try to ignore the pain and push through."
- "Come on; you can walk a little farther."
- "Yesterday, you were doing so well. What happened?"
- "You need to get out more."
- "I've called you several times; why won't you answer?"
- "If you wanted to do it, you would."
- "I miss seeing you in church; where have you been?"
- "You work out more than I do."
- "Why can't you just try?"
- "Here's what you should do…."
- "I heard you went to a concert the other day, so why can't you attend the event now?"

While the symptoms of SPS, such as rigidity and stimulus-triggered painful muscle spasms of predominantly skeletal, trunk, head, or muscles that control the pelvic or shoulder region are grueling to experience,[3]They are less arduous than the communal aspects of living with ICI: specifically, the shortage of support and understanding, while the abundance of unhealthy social interactions and comments proliferates. The latter can aid in your expiry or demise.

Experiencing pain and disappointment can take a heavy toll on one's physical well-being. Constant anger triggers a fight-or-flight response, causing significant changes in heart rate, blood pressure, and immune function. These changes can lead to an increased risk of depression, heart disease, diabetes, and other health issues.[4]

For individuals with disorders impacting their immune system, life can be a constant battle. Their bodies are in a state of heightened inflammation, as evidenced by increased levels of pro-inflammatory cytokines. These powerful proteins, produced by various immune and non-immune cells, are essential for regulating the immune system. Some cytokines act as beacons, alerting the body to invaders and triggering an immune response. Others work to suppress the immune system when necessary. Interestingly, these same cytokines are also elevated during temporary illnesses like the flu. For those with chronic immune disorders, this means that even when their primary condition is being managed, they may still experience symptoms like fatigue, fever, difficulty focusing, body aches, and joint pain—all of which may be hallmarks of a typical flu episode. It's a never-ending cycle of battling against the body's immune system.[5]

Furthermore, for individuals with SPS, an autoimmune disease,[6] the physical burden of chronic anger translates into emotional stress and anxiety, which can exacerbate symptoms, worsening spasms in particular. Emotional stress also increases the aforementioned pro-inflammatory cytokines, which will induce an inflammatory response causing an increase in symptoms and other diseases.[7]

The disappointments of the communal aspects of living with SPS are not just found in the comments made by others, but also in my mind as I desperately try to understand if joy is found in the suffering of others. Few people will easily admit it and for others, it's a difficult truth for many to confess, but there is a certain satisfaction in witnessing the misfortunes of others. The downfall of an arrogant and untalented contestant on a favorite television program, the uncovering of a self-righteous politician's embarrassing vice, the subtle pleasure derived from a supposedly "perfect" friend's minor setback - these moments all elicit a sense of *schadenfreude* that we can't help but savor.[8] As psychologists have delved into this phenomenon, they have revealed that it stems from an aversion to empathy, a fear or unwillingness to truly care because it may require us to take action and make changes in our own lives. It's a defense mechanism, protecting us from the potential discomfort of getting involved in another person's problems.[9]

Numerous published studies have confirmed the idea that caring is a costly endeavor. It requires a significant amount of cognitive effort, which many people are inclined to avoid. When given the opportunity, individuals often opt to shy away from displaying compassion. Research has shown that true compassion demands more than just feeling empathy or remaining neutral; it requires active mental engagement. Therefore, people tend to experience compassion less frequently if they perceive it as mentally draining and burdensome.[10]

While the researcher's insight on the subject may be correct, I find little to no comfort in this awareness. For me, several questions remain:

1. Why can't others see the heavy demands on ICI people trying to cope?
2. Why don't they think about what I go through during the day and at night? For example, the spasms that greet me in the morning and during the night produce spasmsomina.
3. Why don't they understand the stress, anxiety, and physical impact of living with a debilitating disease? The days and nights spent in tears, painful prayer, or meditation, and the unimaginable challenges of standing or walking while in body spasms?

4. Why don't they understand the indescribable fatigue, brain fog, and other side effects, including the lack of good-quality sleep?
5. Why don't they comprehend the in-depth preparation I must undertake to leave the house, such as carrying a rescue bag, medications, medical alert bracelet, and medical resources and being aware of the nearest emergency room? Attending meetings and gatherings and sometimes going to the store requires significant sacrifice and effort.
6. Why don't they understand that living with ICI or SPS will generate a few dark days? They are to be expected. And during this time, rest and personal space are best.
7. Why don't they fathom that I cannot always immediately respond to emails, text messages, or phone calls because I am experiencing pain, spasms, or the side effects of the medication? It's not that I am evading you.
8. Why don't they recognize the sadness I experience when I cannot go somewhere or do what I enjoy because of the disabling symptoms of SPS and the frustration that develops because of the difficulty traveling and making new friends? There is no contentment in becoming incapacitated in public or having spasms related to SPS on a plane which could quickly become an emergency.
9. Why don't they understand how difficult it is to plan for the future, and the stress of living with the forever uncertainty of whether each new day will bring few or no symptoms, or the sorrow that comes with feeling that aspirations or milestones are out of reach?
10. Why don't they understand that when you have a chronic illness, having good support from others is key? (People who have strong social support networks tend to do better long term.)[11]

What are Empathy and Compassion?

While empathy has been explained in various ways over time, there is a consensus that empathy includes understanding others' emotions and/or perspectives, often resonating with others' emotional states. Building on the work of scholars, empathy can be defined as a deep, visceral reaction that mirrors exactly or closely resembles the emotions of another person or what one might anticipate them to feel in a given situation. This response stems from truly comprehending someone else's emotional state or circumstances. For example, you try to imagine yourself in their place to understand what they are feeling or experiencing.[12] Having empathy facilitates prosocial, or "helping" behavior, which originates organically, rather than assistance that has been forced. You feel the desire to want to help, and you understand how the sick individual feels.

Compassion, on the other hand, involves empathy but represents an emotional response in which the perception—real or unreal—of someone or something is suffering and demonstrates a genuine and bona fide desire to provide support. True compassion means not only feeling another's pain but also feeling the weight of another's burden and having an unwavering determination to lift it off their shoulders.[13]

How are empathy and compassion developed, and why do some people lack them? I firmly believe, in large part, that empathy and compassion are developed during early childhood through our environment and the models we observe. I also believe that many people who lack empathy and compassion were nurtured in families and communities where they were encouraged to switch off their feelings for others during early childhood—or as children, they never internalized a connection to their feelings or the emotions of others. To bestow empathy and compassion on others, you must be able to identify situations in your childhood, while developing and growing up, in which you received and observed empathy and compassion in action.

Albert Bandura's pioneering work in social learning theory further helps us understand the benefits of observing the expression of empathy and compassion during early development or childhood. He suggests that observation and modeling are primary roles in how and why people learn. Learning is not only the result of our direct experience with the environment but can occur simply by observing others' behavior. He explains that most of our actions as humans are learned by observing others and imitating their behavior. Through this process, we develop a framework for performing new tasks and actions, which we can then use as a guide in the future.[14] In simple terms, we observe other people's behavior and assimilate and imitate the observed behavior. Finally, we are more likely to imitate behavior modeled by people we perceive as similar to ourselves. People we perceive to be akin to ourselves include but are not limited to parents, siblings, and community members. Additionally, people tend to feel the most empathy for others who share similarities with them, whether it be physical appearance, past experiences of hardship, or a common purpose.[15]

Although social learning is a major contributor to how people learn, it does not tell the complete story. This is especially true regarding the development of empathy and compassion. A study published in 2018 suggests that how empathic we are is not just a result of our upbringing and experience, but partly a result of our genes.[16] The debate about how we develop and learn continues.

Over the past few years, I've enjoyed reconnecting with an early childhood friend, Betty, and her family. Her brother was my first mentor, protector, teacher, and friend. He is now deceased. Since relinking with Betty—mainly once she learned about the SPS diagnosis—she has connected with me weekly to check-in. Sometimes, she shares a funny situation, chit-chats about social issues, asks questions about the family, or sees if I need anything. She expresses that her love and support are unwavering. Betty is also part of a close-knit group that practices prosocial behavior with one another and within their extended family. Recently, I asked Betty what encourages her to ask how she could help show compassionate empathy. How is it that she is in a community of friends who share in expressing prosocial behaviors? Betty spoke with her friends, and they provided the following statements:

1. "We were taught that if you can help someone in need, do it cheerfully."
2. "You have to be forgiving. Don't block your blessings when you're mistreated."
3. "No matter what the kids did wrong, mom never turned them away. Instead, she gave, raised her kids, and continued to pray and trust in God."
4. "I got involved in a program called Off the Street Club, which provided activities and tutoring to the neighborhood. I learned how to crochet and made money selling hats and scarves in grammar school."
5. "We grew up in a community where they had block club parties, and kids played jump rope, hide, and seek, softball, red light, green light, board games, et cetera. So many of the relationships and social interactions remain today."
6. "We were taught not to judge and to be humble, trustworthy, independent, protective, loving, and

dependable. Neighbors were family and would go to the store for the elders. The kids in the neighborhood learned to lose gracefully when playing games. They were taught not to misuse anyone and not to hurt others intentionally. Ask for forgiveness if you're wrong. Be forgiving. Praise those who need it. Feed those who are hungry. Don't be negative."

7. "I was taught to respect people who are in authority."
8. "The church had summer-long programs that taught us many valuable lessons about helping those in need."
9. "As a young child, I attended nursing homes with my pastor and learned how to care for the sick."
10. "Currently, I am the full-time caregiver for my mother."

Based on their comments, Betty and her friends had a rich opportunity to practice empathy and compassion. Their childhood was the catalytic agent, and they internalized their observations, emotions, and encounters.

Betty is not the only friend who expresses empathy and compassion. Over the last few years, I've had an opportunity to provide emotional support, health education, and resources to a group of people from the Horn of Africa. And although the war in their country is very heartbreaking, they realize that a part of the experience of being human is feeling empathy and compassion for others. The group leader connects with me often to see how I am doing.

The answer to why some people lack empathy and compassion can be explained by having not experienced or observed empathy and compassion during childhood, including a lack of encouragement and education on connecting your feelings with prosocial behavior. "Where the mind goes, behavior will follow."[17]

How to Cope When Empathy and Compassion Are Not Present

While I believe being happy, compassionate, and empathic to others is essential, I also grew up in the same neighborhood, community environment, and family structure as Betty and her friends. I attended Dr. Martin Luther King Jr. Boys and Girls Club[18] and social and sports programs sponsored by Marillac Social Center[19] and witnessed neighbors helping neighbors. These childhood encounters fostered in me a level of caring and sensitivity for others. Contacting my friends only when I have a need or a question, would never be acceptable. I do not see how a friendship can be maintained when interaction only occurs in person. If I know that a family member or a friend is sick, I routinely reach out to them. A simple note to say, "Hey, I am thinking about you today," goes a long way to promote caring. Perhaps, this is why exhibiting prosocial behavior is so important to me.

However, being content around people lacking empathy and compassion can be very challenging. But despite the circumstances, isolating is not a healthy option. Love and compassion are essential for our existence, not mere luxuries. Without them, we are doomed to self-destruction.[20] It hurts when concern is absent. It can be a very nerve-racking condition. Unfortunately, despite signaling to family, friends, and the public that you are struggling with an ICI, your best efforts may fall short. Understanding that your family and friends cannot represent your support system's totality will help you focus on managing your health instead of controlling the irritability interpersonal relationships can bring.

Here are a few suggestions to help alter your mindset:

1. Never stop being compassionately empathic to others despite the lack of reciprocity. The more we care and help others, the greater our sense of well-being. Unfortunately, this life is full of disappointments; thus, we will encounter problems. But if we lose hope and become depressed, unhappy, and discouraged, we will hamper our immune system, increase ICI symptoms, and perhaps develop other diseases. You can choose to be the missing model they have yet to observe.
2. Make your health the priority, not trying to fix others. Remember, you don't have to agree with how other people behave, and nothing you say or do will change them.
3. Do not take it personally: Remind yourself that it is not your fault. Most likely, their lack of empathy and compassion results from poor childhood exposure and is usually unintentional. Also, some people who cannot show empathy or compassion to others may suffer from mental health disorders such as narcissistic personality disorder (NPD), Machiavellianism, sociopathy or antisocial personality disorder, borderline personality disorder (BPD), alexithymia, or autism.[21]Additionally, some adults act puerilely and are developmentally delayed in the management of their emotions which results in adhering to only their needs. Individuals who have been diagnosed with immature personality disorder often exhibit this behavior.[22]
4. You don't have to take abuse. Instead, learn to set boundaries and remove toxic people from your life.

5. Seek professional help. Dealing with people who lack empathy can be an incredibly isolating experience. And struggling alone isn't the answer to getting through difficult times. Seeking help provides the best opportunity to resolve your challenges while establishing that supportive resource, especially when you need assistance the most.

LEARNING AND DISCUSSION: HOW CAN THOSE WHO CARE HELP?

Practice Active Listening What is active listening?

It involves absorbing the information someone shares with you and responding with thoughtful questions and attentive, reflective body language to show that you are making it clear that you truly hear another person and that they are understood. Think of it as engaging in empathetic conversation where one truly listens and builds a strong connection with another.

When someone opens up to you about their chronic illness, it is crucial to engage in actively listening as they share things with you about their illness. Active listening also entails showing those with a chronic illness that you really do care by signaling to them that you've heard how the illness impacts their life. Chiefly, be willing to learn how sickness affects their daily living by encouraging them to share their perspectives and insights on subjects related to their care.

One of the most effective ways to do this is by refraining from offering unsolicited opinions, even if they are well-intentioned. This, too, includes refraining from equating one's experiences to those facing health challenges. During those verbal exchanges, you may try to provide comfort, empathize with them, and let them know you understand what is being experienced by discussing a similar experience. Don't! As active listeners, it is essential to remember that even though you may have experienced something similar to what the person is describing, the two experiences will never be the same, especially when accounting for sociocultural elements within our environment, such as cultural norms and gender roles, in addition to the diverse ways in which people make connections between newly acquired information and their existing knowledge. The latter is especially true when the listener is from a different cultural group than the person they seek to assist.[23]

Often, when I share my diagnosis of SPS with others and I explain the symptoms, they will usually talk about their experience (s) with spasms in an attempt to relate to my situation. I understand their desire to be empathic; it's appreciated but also a missed opportunity. Again, no two tribulations or woes are the same, even if the person that I am referring to has been diagnosed with SPS.

Furthermore, being conscious of and attentive to the words and the language we use in our conversations can significantly impact the quality of our relationships. It's important not to dismiss someone's feelings or discredit their thoughts with phrases like:

- "You shouldn't let it bring you down;"
- "You don't have to feel overwhelmed or stuck, because there is always a way to move forward."
- "It's not as terrible as you think; there's no need to dwell on it."
- "It's time to move on and leave this behind, you're blowing it out of proportion."
- "You have a tendency to take things too personally and give them more significance than necessary."
- "Think only good thoughts."
- "Everyone must endure some rainy days; we all face our health struggles."
- "We all go through aches and pains, we all get tired, it's just a part of life."

- "Don't worry, you'll be okay."
- "It is what it is."

Remember that generally, people will feel more open to sharing what they need with people they know can be trusted and respectful. By practicing active listening, you can make communicating easier with someone whose health is compromised.

15 Encouraging Phrases to Offer Someone Battling a Chronic Illness

1. "I know that living with Stiff Person Syndrome can be incredibly challenging. I cannot fully comprehend the difficulties you face, but please know that I am here for you and will support you through your journey."
2. "If your plans need to change, don't feel bad, just let me know and I'll adjust; accordingly, I got you."
3. "I'm about to grab a glass of wine; would you like a glass, red or white?"
4. "How are you feeling today?"
5. "I'm thinking about you."
6. "It seems like you're going through a tough time. What can I do to help and support you in this moment?"
7. "If you need someone to talk to, I am here to listen."
8. "Let's set a time to talk regularly. We don't always have to discuss health issues."
9. "I believe you."
10. "I wanted to reach out and see how you're doing. I hope you know that I love and care about you deeply; and miss having you around."

11. "I'm saddened by the news of your diagnosis. If you ever need someone to talk to, I am here for you and am willing to lend an ear."
12. "I have a fantastic restaurant in mind, would you like me to bring you some food today? Is there anything specific you would like to order?"
13. "Let's divide and conquer our shopping trip. We can divide the grocery list and meet at the produce section. You pick your items first."
14. "I read up on Stiff-Person Syndrome and the information was very interesting. I'd like to share it with you and hear your thoughts. Is that okay?"
15. "How do you take care of yourself on days when you're not feeling your best? And what activities do you enjoy doing on the days when things are going better?"

If you live with Stiff Person Syndrome or another chronic illness, what are some phrases you wish you heard more often from family and friends?

1. ______________________________
2. ______________________________
3. ______________________________
4. ______________________________
5. ______________________________
6. ______________________________
7. ______________________________

8. ____

9. ____

10. ____

As previously mentioned, people in general can be ultra-insensitive because of childhood experiences that influenced their development of empathy and compassion. How about you? What were your parents and community like when you were a child? What childhood experiences helped shape how you show empathy and compassion?

List ten valuable lessons from childhood that influenced how you show empathy and compassion today.

1. ____

2. ____

3. ____

4. ____

5. ____

6. ____

7. ____

8. ____

9. ____

10. ____

Lastly, if you are a caregiver or provide support to a loved one or friend with a chronic illness, don't forget to take care of yourself, too, so you can offer the best assistance possible. You might consider finding out more about the national organizations listed below to see if they can meet your specific needs and support you in the ways you need it most.

The Well Spouse Association
https://wellspouse.org/

The WSA (Well Spouse Association) is a non-profit organization with a nationwide reach, providing resources, and support to spouses and partners of those with chronic illnesses or disabilities. They strive to advocate for and attend to the specific needs of caregivers in these situations; while also bringing attention to the challenges they face through education initiatives aimed at healthcare professionals and the public.

The EPIC Foundation
Empowering People with Invisible Chronic Illness
https://epictogether.org/

The EPIC Foundation is a registered 501(c)(3) non-profit organization that offers assistance, representation, and resources to individuals impacted by chronic illnesses. Their team of qualified psychologists provides a range of services to aid patients and their caregivers, including emotional support and practical tools to help them flourish in the face of prolonged illnesses.

The National Alliance for Caregiving
https://www.caregiving.org/

The National Alliance for Caregiving is a collaboration of non-profit organizations with a shared goal of creating a society that recognizes, supports, and empowers family caregivers to succeed in their roles at home, work, and in life. Their objective is to form alliances through research, advocacy, and innovation to improve the lives of family caregivers.

CHAPTER THREE

TURNING TO CANNABIS

I was initially reluctant to try cannabis as a treatment regimen. After years of training to become a clinical neuropsychologist, and teaching courses in behavioral medicine, including psychopharmacology, I was aware of the risks associated with cannabis. Thoughts of becoming a "junkie," losing control of my mind, and becoming addicted were significant concerns. But those fears quickly dissipated after hearing these words from my medical team consisting of primary care, neurology, pain management, and rheumatology, all of whom worked very hard to help me to be able to function: "Dr. Scott, I don't know what else can be done for you. You have failed all the treatments, and the spasms are still happening. I feel very bad for you. We can try biologics. There is nothing else that I can do for you. I have no other recommendations."

Muscle spasms are usually treated with pain relievers (analgesics), anti-inflammatory drugs, anti-anxiety medication, muscle relaxers, or, in some cases, biologics or Botulinum toxin. However, not only did these medications produce intolerable side effects, such as nausea and elevated liver enzymes, but they were ineffective. This led me to turn to cannabis as my last hope for a muscle spasm treatment.

In early 2019, I began re-educating myself about the medical benefits of cannabis with the goal of leaving no stone unturned as I desperately searched for a treatment to help alleviate the spasms. By this time, I was battling reading, exploring, and learning while coping with spasms, pain, stiffness, and the side effects of Valium. As mentioned, Stiff Person Syndrome (SPS) is a rare central nervous system disorder. It's a neurological disease characterized by rigidity and painful, stimulus-triggered muscle spasms of predominantly the skeletal system, trunk, head, or muscles that control the pelvic or shoulder region. The spasms can be so severe that the experience can be like the feeling of bones breaking or joints dislocating. The spasms can dislocate joints and even break bones.[1] The most common areas that SPS affects my body are the feet, hands, arms, abdomen, thighs, calves, shin, and sometimes, the throat. There are at least four variants of SPS that have been described, affecting sufferers in different ways.[2]

After an exhaustive review of the literature, including reading countless patients' stories of success with cannabis as a treatment for pain and muscle stiffness, I approached my primary care doctor. I asked if he would support my use of medical cannabis. It was my last hope of treatment because there were no other options.

In late 2019, I received a state medical cannabis registration card and began discovering its benefits. But, unfortunately, it took me three months of trial and error to find the right combination, strain, and method to relieve the spasms, decrease their intensity, and decrease their likelihood of persistently occurring.

About Medical Cannabis

Historical evidence suggests that the herb may have been used for medicinal purposes in the region as far back as 2000 BC. It was believed to have potential benefits for glaucoma, cataracts, hemorrhoids, vaginal bleeding, and even cancer. Surprisingly, when the mummy of Pharaoh Ramesses II was discovered and examined in 1881, residues of cannabis were found within his corpse. Further examinations of other mummies have also revealed the presence of cannabis, solidifying the belief that it was a common part of ancient Egyptian culture.[3]

Cannabis Sativa has been known for its medicinal benefits for more than two millennia.[4] It was available as a licensed medicine in the United States for about a century before the American Medical Association removed it from the 12th edition of the U.S. Pharmacopeia.[5]

Cannabis or Marijuana?

It's not surprising to often hear the words "cannabis" and "marijuana" used synonymously, but this is a misunderstanding because they don't mean the same thing. Instead, "cannabis" refers to all products derived from Cannabis Sativa and, more distinctly, to the genus or family of plants, including Cannabis Indica, Cannabis Sativa, and Cannabis Ruderalis. The cannabis plant contains about 540 chemical substances.

The word "marijuana" refers to parts of or products from the plant Cannabis Sativa that contain substantial amounts of tetrahydrocannabinol (THC). THC is the substance that's noted for the effects of marijuana on a person's cognitive and mental state. Some cannabis plants contain minimal THC. The term marijuana also carries a negative, racist connotation, geared towards helping to stigmatize and criminalize users while combating the so-called "war on drugs."[6]

Medical Cannabis for Muscle Spasms

Medical cannabis is very effective in relieving SPS spasms of varying severity and intensity. This is likely the case because several cannabinoids in cannabis are identified as relieving spasmodic symptoms, as shown in the clinical literature involving patients who experience chronic and painful spasms.[7]

Below are a few examples of formal studies showing that cannabis relieves muscle spasms. However, any time a supplement, product, or medication is consumed and used; it is wise to do your research and consult medical professionals to make informed and safe choices.

- Treated with THC-CBD oromucosal spray, improvement was verified in the eight dimensions of the scale of the SF-36 quality of life questionnaire. Cannabis derivatives therapy for a seronegative Stiff Person Syndrome: a case report[8]
- Reported benefits of cannabis use for muscle spasms.[9]
- Efficacy and safety of medical marijuana in selected neurologic disorders[10]
- California research shows pot can ease muscle spasms.[11]
- A study published by the Journal of Neuroimmune Pharmacology reported chemicals found in cannabis are encouraging for people suffering from severe or persistent muscle spasms.[12]
- There is a large amount of evidence to support the view that the psychoactive ingredient in cannabis, delta9-tetrahydrocannabinol (delta9-THC), and cannabinoids in general, can reduce muscle spasticity and pain under some circumstances.[13]
- Medical cannabis is an accepted therapy for muscle spastic disorders.[14]

- Significant improvement in spasticity and quality of life. Medical Cannabis for Pediatric Moderate to Severe Complex Motor Disorders.[15]
- Results confirm the effectiveness of THC: CBD therapy to reduce treatment-resistant MS spasticity and sustain improvement for 18 months.[16]
- Cannabis Extract Improves Spasticity Without Increasing Weakness in Patients With MS.

As indicated in the studies above and the literature, the cannabinoids in cannabis that are anti-spasmodic are THC, cannabidiol (CBD), cannabigerol (CBG), and tetrahydrocannabinolic acid (THCA). But more than 100 other cannabinoids have been identified.

The main cannabinoids, THC and CBD, are essential for relieving muscle spasms. They are also the most researched and studied. These are the most critical cannabinoids when choosing a strain or product to relieve muscle spasms. The main difference between the two cannabinoids is that THC has psychoactive effects, meaning it makes a person 'high,' whereas CBD is thought to have an anti-psychoactive effect that controls or moderates the 'high' caused by the THC. CBD is also believed to reduce some of the other unwanted effects people can experience from THC, such as anxiety.[17]

Benefits of THC

- Pain Relief
- Eases Nausea & Vomiting
- Increases Appetite
- Effective Sleep Aid

- Helps Treat Post Traumatic Stress Disorder
- Antibacterial
- Antioxidant
- Anti-inflammatory
- Bronchodilator
- Potential anti-tumor agent
- Muscle relaxant
- Anticonvulsant

Benefits of CBD

- Treatment for Epilepsy
- Pain Relief
- Relieve Pain and Inflammation Associated with Arthritis
- Relieve Anxiety
- Decrease Symptoms of Depression
- Enhance Sleep
- Relieve Symptoms of Parkinson's Disease

Why Does Cannabis Work?

The reason why cannabis is so beneficial to our health is because of our endocannabinoid system (ECS). The ECS is a biological network that lies within our bodies in areas such as the brain (central nervous system), immune cells, and connective tissue. It's responsible for keeping us in balance. The ECS is the gatekeeper or the control system that assists our body in staying healthy. They are neurotransmitters. Neurotransmitters are chemical messengers in the body that send signals between cells. For example, the ECS sends signals between cells to regulate pain, inflammation, cardiovascular, gastrointestinal, respiratory systems, metabolism, and immunity. It also helps to control our memory, mood, appetite, and sleep.

The cannabinoids in cannabis mimic ECS by interacting and signaling cells in the same way, thus, producing responses to regulate pain and impact our appetite, sleep, and other functions.

Cannabis Strains

You should also consider the type of strain or product when using cannabis. Indica and Indica-dominant hybrid strains are known for their full-body sedative effects. It's ideal for those looking to relax or require a better night's sleep. Many people suffering from anxiety, pain, or muscle spasms also turn to Indica strains because it helps them pull through by allowing them to sleep and rest more easily.

Sativa and Sativa-dominant hybrid strains and products are more invigorating and stimulating than the Indica strains. Individuals use these strains to feel more social, physically active, energetic, and creative. Sativa is the best choice for daytime relief of symptoms.

Presently, there is a quarrel as to whether Sativa and Indica are two different strains.[18]

While recognizing that there are many benefits of using THC or CBD alone, after the first three months of cannabis use, I found that the most effective ratio of cannabis use was 50/50 Sativa/Indica hybrid 1:1 THC to CBD or a 1:1 Indica. This 1:1 ratio is also consistent with most studies regarding cannabis and the relief of muscle spasms. The general rule in discovering which ratio or strain of cannabis will be most beneficial to you is to "start low and go slow."

Because THC and CBD properties also reduce pain, this is an added benefit for relieving the debilitating component of spasms associated with SPS, and using them in combination provides excellent relief.

I use gummies, chocolates, candies (edibles), or a tincture to get me through the night. While they have a slower onset of action, they tend to get me through the night pain and spasm-free. I can generally get about six hours of relief using these products. However, if I require immediate comfort, I vape. Vaping's onset of action is usually within fifteen minutes, but since it has a shorter half-life, the relief lasts between one and three hours.

What is half-life? In general, half-life refers to how long it takes for half of a single dose of a drug to leave the body. It helps to explain how long a medication will stay in human systems, and it is usually affected by factors like the route of administration, dosage, age, and frequency of use. Picking the suitable intake method is a matter of preference and will depend on your circumstances and symptoms.

Conclusion

As mentioned, the basic rule to follow when learning how to dose cannabis is to start low with small doses and go slow, gradually increasing in small amounts until you find an appropriate dose that relieves symptoms without unwanted side effects. Finding the right dose and strain to relieve your symptoms will take time. I recommend keeping a journal, noting the time of day, route of administration (the way that a drug is placed into the body), the amount used, strain, the onset of action (how long it took to feel the effects), feelings, symptoms relieved, and side effects.

My goal of easing and slowing the occurrence of spasms associated with SPS has been accomplished with medical cannabis, but not without experiencing side effects such as lethargy, mental dullness, and a temporary decrease in my desire to engage in challenging or demanding tasks that might require too much effort. Cannabis is not a cure for SPS or associated spasms, but it has helped considerably. And, the benefits have outweighed the cost. The spasms are at times better controlled, and there are no signs of cannabis toxicity damage, to the liver or kidney after four years of moderate to heavy use.

Cannabis is a versatile medicine. But, to use it effectively to relieve muscle spasms associated with SPS, you should be knowledgeable about strain types, THC and CBD ratios, dosing, and ways to use the medicine.

LEARNING AND DISCUSSION: USING CANNABIS

As medical cannabis becomes an option for the treatment of SPS and many chronic conditions, it is of the utmost importance to be well-informed about what is needed and required to use it legally and safely.

Below is the strategy I undertook in pursuit of starting the journey of using medical cannabis. I hope that the revelation of my approach will provide you with the necessary insights and road map to obtain the support of your medical team to use medical cannabis.

If I Am Interested In Using Medical Cannabis, What Steps Should I Take?

- **Research Your State Laws Regarding Cannabis Use.**

One starting point is to research your state's laws to determine the legality of adult use of medical cannabis. Despite its classification as an illegal substance on the federal level, alongside drugs like heroin and LSD that carry criminal penalties for possession, several states have chosen to legalize cannabis for both recreational and medical purposes. But on May 16, 2024, the United States Department of Justice (DOJ), also known as the Justice Department, announced that it was taking major steps to reclassify cannabis. This shift was fueled by the President of the United States (POTUS) directive on August 20, 2023, to the Department of Health and Human Services (HHS) to make a scheduling recommendation for cannabis to be given to the Department of Drug Enforcement Agency (DEA). This change in approach indicates that cannabis will probably be moved from Schedule I to Schedule III on the controlled substance list, meaning it will be subject to less stringent regulations.[19]

Additionally, before using cannabis, it is also crucial to consider your employer's drug policy, including drug testing, and determine, if appropriate, whether your industry or profession has regulations or strict standards regarding cannabis use. If you have concerns or need further guidance, seek legal counsel.

- **Learn About Cannabis.**

Before diving into cannabis use, it's very important to educate oneself about the herbal plant and its effects. This will provide a more comprehensive understanding of the potential health effects and risks associated with its use, including any immediate and long lasting impacts on physical well-being, mental state, and cognitive abilities.

As I previously mentioned, being well-informed about cannabis can also aid in making responsible decisions regarding its consumption and use. Through education, individuals are equipped with key information, ultimately allowing them to make choices that align with their personal beliefs and aspirations.

One of the most prudent ways people educate themselves is by using the internet, especially social media, and website pages. There is a plethora of information about cannabis on the internet. However, despite the abundance of data available, a wealth of misinformation has also proliferated on social media sites and the internet, causing widespread misunderstandings. Misinformation on social media is of particular concern because of its accessibility and immediate, immeasurable reach, which can lead to significant consequences for the health and medical care of those who adhere to the assertions. It is worthwhile to carefully consider the sources you read and believe when it comes to cannabis. This herbal plant is not a cure-all miracle solution. While some claims about its medicinal benefits are supported by robust clinical evidence, many other testimonies lack rigorous scientific backing. There remains disagreement among cannabis experts on how safe it is and how well it works.[20] As researchers continue to study cannabis, it is essential to rely on medical advice from your healthcare provider rather than using cannabis as a substitute for more appropriate treatment.

- **Speak With Your Doctor.**

Talking with your doctor about how medical cannabis can fit into your overall treatment plan can be intimidating. You may be hesitant to talk with your doctor for various reasons. One reason that many Black/African American, Indigenous, Latino, Latinx, or Hispanic individuals might be less apt to share about their desire to use medical cannabis is for fear of impending microaggressions and reduced quality of care.

Without question, historically, the United States of America's healthcare system has not shown enmeshment of respect, social sensitivity, an inescapable social responsibility, nor a profound concern for all human beings. It has rather created medical racism and reinforced it, even today.[21]

While a breakthrough in America's conscience concerning healthcare yet exists, it's understandable you might be resistant to conversing with your doctor about consuming cannabis; however, it is critical to discuss your desire to use cannabis. Cannabis is a powerful substance that can interfere or interact with other medicines, prescription drugs, herbs, remedies, and even anesthesia. Your doctor will know the medications that cannabis may interact with and help you to avoid a potentially dangerous outcome. Likewise, if you see more than one doctor and have been prescribed or are using cannabis, it is necessary to share with each of them that you are using cannabis and allow them to determine if there is a cause for concern.

Currently, hundreds of drugs may cause a drug interaction when used with cannabis.[22] To avoid drug interactions, it will require you to be able to honestly and openly discuss cannabis use with your healthcare providers.

- What is a drug interaction? A drug interaction occurs when medications react with each other, particular food, and drinks, or even pre-existing medical conditions, leading to unforeseen, unwelcome, and possibly dangerous side effects. It is crucial to understand possible drug interactions to avoid any adverse consequences.

In preparation for meeting with your doctor to talk about using medical cannabis consider discussing these topics and writing down the answers so that you can better understand how to use cannabis safely.

- Explain why you want to use cannabis and what you'd like the outcome to be.
- Will cannabis help my medical condition?
- Does my medical condition qualify for cannabis treatment in my state?
- Should I stop using cannabis when I feel better?
- What are the side effects of cannabis?
- What should I do if I have a side effect?
- Are there foods, drinks (including alcohol), other medicines, or activities to avoid while I am using cannabis?
- Are there any tests I need while I am using cannabis?
- Can I become addicted to cannabis?

What To Do If My Doctor Says "NO" To Using Medical Cannabis?

After diligently conducting research and having honest discussions with your doctor, there is still a chance that they may have reservations about recommending medical cannabis for various reasons. Their decision to say no may have nothing to do with whether cannabis can be of help to you. Many healthcare professionals are not very knowledgeable or open-minded about alternative forms of medicine such as medical cannabis.

Nevertheless, this is a matter of your health, and your well-being. Don't let one hesitant opinion discourage you from exploring all of your options for finding relief and managing your health. With determination and perseverance, you can find a healthcare provider who shares your vision for holistic healing.

Finally, keep in mind that your primary care doctor does not issue prescriptions for medical cannabis. Instead, they certify that a patient has a qualifying medical condition for its use. Once you have successfully obtained your certification, you are now eligible to apply for a medical cannabis card through your state's official program.

Medical Cannabis Journal

Cannabinoid percentage **Strain**

THC %			Indica	YES NO
CBD %			Sativa	YES NO
CBG %			Hybrid	YES NO

Route used **Product type**

Eaten		Concentrates/Dabs	
Inhaled/Smoked		Edibles	
Oral		Flower	
Rectally		Tinctures	
Tropical		Topicals	
Sublingual (place underneath the tongue)		Vape	

Amount of cannabis used

Desired Symptom Relief: Check all that apply

Chronic Pain Relief		Improve Sleep	
Alleviate Spasms		Decrease Depression	
Seizure Control		Reduce Anxiety	
Reduction of Inflammation		Improve Symptoms of Post Traumatic Stress Disorder	
Control Vomiting		Relaxation	
Increase Appetite		Relieve Nausea	

How long before you felt its effects?	How long before the effects ended?

Was it effective?

Side effects: Check all that apply

Altered senses		Impaired memory and thinking	
An altered sense of time and space		Increased appetite	
Confusion and disorientation		Increased heart rate	
Dizziness		Panic attacks/increased anxiety	
Drug interaction		Paranoia	
Dry mouth		Poor muscle coordination	
Exhilaration/high		Red eyes	

Focus		Relaxation or sleepiness	
Foggy		Sex and intimacy	
Food interaction		Slower reaction times	
Hallucinations/ delusions		Spiritual	

Notes:

Medical Cannabis Resources:

The Academy of Medical Cannabis
https://learn.taomc.org/our-courses/

Center for Medicinal Cannabis Research
https://www.cmcr.ucsd.edu/index.php

Multidisciplinary Center for Cannabinoid Research
https://cannabinoids.huji.ac.il/people/raphael-mechoulam

The Scientist
https://youtu.be/5BGS5JzLlvs

Prof. Raphael Mechoulam-Medical Cannabis Complete Interview
https://youtu.be/sD1ZF0dE5nw

Grotenhermen, Franjo & Russo, Ethan. (2002). Cannabis and Cannabinoids

Pharmacology, Toxicology, and Therapeutic Potential.

Ditchfield, Jeff & Thomas, Mel. (2014). The Medical Cannabis Guidebook: The Definitive Guide to Using and Growing Medicinal Marijuana

Whiteley, Nishi. (2016). Chronic Relief: A Guide to Cannabis for the Terminally and Chronically Ill.

CHAPTER FOUR

COPING WITH THE PAIN, STIFFNESS, AND SPASMS OF STIFF PERSON SYNDROME

The onset of the spasms of Stiff Person Syndrome (SPS) can be unpredictable yet constant. You kind of remember what a morning stretch before arising from a night slumber was like, or the feeling of a cough, a sneeze, or even a joyful laugh before the diagnosis happened. Now those routine and reflexive spasms-free days are a distant memory. Who would have guessed that a morning stretch, a shave, or stepping into a hot shower could alter your life? You are left trying to figure out how to live this way and find happiness.

Living and thriving with SPS demands that you gear up for daily and moment-to-moment life adjustments. Many of the required adjustments involve your thoughts, while others are physical. On some days you can do more than on others, but each day you must determine in your heart and mind that you will do something to help improve the quality of your life and add joy to the day. I expect every day to exercise, relax, eat a healthy, whole-food, plant-based diet, and contribute to the life of someone who is in need. While the spasms may change the time of the day the activities take place, and though I may not be able to do the same activities I once did, spasms will never change the occurrence of them.

Coping with Stiff Person Syndrome starts as an act of your will fueled by the mind. This leads to behavior changes that produce benefits. Where the mind goes, the behavior will follow.

What I Have Learned Through This Opportunity

There is no doubt that discomfort, pain, struggle, and coping with adversities can be a great teacher. Without question, many of the most painful endeavors can help to enhance our lives.

Here are a couple of insights that I have gained:

1. **"Give Thanks For A Little And You Will Find A Lot."**
   - Learning to be thankful and finding gratitude in life is associated with several mental and physical health benefits. Demonstrating thankfulness is the catalyst for finding joy, peace, and fulfillment in life. Research suggests that gratitude may be associated with many benefits for individuals, including better physical and psychological health, increased happiness and life satisfaction, decreased materialism, and more.[1]
     - A handful of reports suggest that more grateful people may be healthier, and others suggest that scientifically designed practices to increase gratitude can also improve people's health and encourage them to adopt healthier habits.
     - Many more findings have examined possible connections between gratitude and various elements of psychological well-being. In general, more grateful

people are happier, more satisfied with their lives, less materialistic, and less likely to suffer from burnout.

  - Additionally, some studies have found that gratitude practices, like keeping a "gratitude journal" or writing a letter of gratitude, can increase people's happiness and overall positive mood.
  - Gratitude may also benefit people with various medical and psychological challenges. For example, one study found that more grateful cardiac patients reported better sleep, less fatigue, and lower levels of cellular inflammation, and another found that heart failure patients who kept a gratitude journal for eight weeks were more grateful and had reduced signs of inflammation afterward.
  - Several articles have found that more grateful people experience less depression and are more resilient following traumatic events. Other data suggest that gratitude may live up to its reputation as the most important virtue of all by nurturing the cultivation of additional moral qualities such as patience, humility, and wisdom.[2] So even if you are having discomfort, pain, or spasms, or are discouraged, there are things that you can be thankful and grateful for.

- **Start A Gratitude Journal.** Gratitude journals are great ways to make thankfulness a part of your daily routine.
- **Find Daily Gratitude Quotes.** Make a calendar with daily, weekly, or monthly gratitude quotes you want to put into practice. Quotes are great resources to inspire us and help us reflect on the good in life.

- **Send Thank You Notes or Cards.** Whether it's for a birthday gift, Christmas present, graduation gift, or for something they helped you with–thank you cards make a big impact. Not only do they let the other person know how much they're appreciated, but they also help you practice gratitude.
- **Do Something Kind for Another Person.** This is a way to show that you are grateful.
- **Pay Attention to the Small Things.** Focus on the little things in your life that bring you joy and peace.
- **Practice Meditation and Prayer.** This helps you intentionally focus on giving thanks.

2. Emotions Are Not Your Guide.

Many people consider pain to be purely physical, but pain is defined as an unpleasant subjective experience with a sensory and an emotional component.[3] Indeed, mental, or better yet, psychological health, especially anxiety, depression, and anger, are highly prevalent in people with chronic pain.[4]

Emotional health includes taking our feelings seriously and not suppressing them. But it does not end here. Emotions are beneficial to help provide support, encouragement, and motivation to assist us in reaching our goals in life. However, they are not meant to tell us whether our goals are healthy and beneficial or whether they represent a useful purpose. Additionally, dwelling on these emotions can cause stress, which has been shown to worsen pain.

Emotions cannot tell us if our decisions are right or wrong. Our principles, morals, and values serve that purpose. But while emotions are limited in scope, they are essential, and it's important that they are not ignored. Ignoring emotions can encourage the denial of the progression of illness and the acknowledgment that we are unhappy. For the chronically ill, this denial often translates into pain.

Emotions and the Chronic Pain Cycle

The experience of pain is complex and influenced by a myriad of factors including emotions. The cycle of pain and emotions are intimately intertwined, each feeding into the other in a continuous loop. Emotions can have a direct impact on physical changes within the body, as seen when anxious or angry individuals experience muscle tension that can contribute to increased levels of pain. This can be especially challenging for anyone who may feel judged for expressing their intense emotions during treatment. However, maintaining a strong belief in one's resilience and ability to adapt can greatly improve overall mood and well-being, providing a glimmer of hope amidst the overwhelming weight of pain and emotions.[5]

While it's important to acknowledge painful emotions, it's more important to understand their purpose. Yes, acknowledge the emotion, but more essentially decide whether the emotion is pushing you in a helpful direction (toward life) or toward an unhealthy direction (away from humanity). Once you decide your direction, the emotions will fall into line and help to support your directional goal.

Don't be afraid to take control of your emotions. You have them for a reason. Allow yourself to feel them, just don't allow them to guide you and your decisions. Painful feelings are natural and completely normal. Encourage good emotional health by feeling them, and then urge yourself to move on, not clinging to these emotions or the corresponding thought patterns.

3. Meditate.

When your chronic pain persists after you've tried conventional treatments, it may be worth a look at meditation. Even if you're skeptical, you may find a type of meditation that helps you. Meditation can help relieve chronic pain by triggering the release of endorphins, your body's natural painkillers.[6] A more recent study from 2020 found that participants with chronic pain who undertook an 8-week mindfulness-based stress reduction course experienced a reduction in depression and pain scores at the end of the 8-week session.[7] Meditation may also boost your pain tolerance by lowering cortisol, a leading cause of inflammation, according to a 2013 study involving 30 second-year medical students.[8] By promoting the release of endorphins, your body's natural painkillers, meditation can provide relief for persistent pain. It may also decrease stress and depression while increasing your tolerance for pain by reducing levels of cortisol, a key contributor to inflammation. As a complementary treatment, meditation can be used alongside conventional methods of managing pain, such as medication, and therapy.[9]

In the stillness of meditation, one can release oneself from the chains of negative emotions that promote and enhance pain, while discovering our inner strength. It is a conscious choice to let go of the pain that can consume us, and instead honor our lives and journey. We must recognize our courage and worthiness of love as we embark on a path toward healing, guided by hope.[10] In the silence of meditation, with each breath, we open our hearts and minds to our pain. But in doing so, we weaken its grip on us, bit by bit, and reduce the tendency of the brain to anticipate it. And with each practice, it becomes easier to reclaim and restore our well-being. As the pain arises again in the future, we approach it with the same mindset—acknowledging it, but not allowing it to overpower us. Through dedication and perseverance, we can break free from its hold and find peace within ourselves. Researchers have also found that meditation helps people live more in the moment, which reduces the tendency of the brain to anticipate pain.[11]

I was first introduced to the benefits of mindfulness, meditation, relaxation, and breathing exercises during clinical training in graduate school. As a clinical psychology student, I helped clients attain positive coping mechanisms to prevent or alleviate stress symptoms and stress-related disorders through mindfulness and meditation. Yet, it was through my long-standing relationship and time spent practicing tai chi with the monks and kung fu masters from the Shaolin Temple in Henan Province, China, that I began to use mindfulness and meditation for my self-care. I practice meditation exercises daily, and the regularity of using these techniques has helped lessen many negative and unwanted thoughts about spasms, stiffness, and pain.

4. Educate Yourself.

Having Stiff Person Syndrome becomes a full-time job. Knowing as much as possible about the disease helps you understand what to expect and how to prepare. It's important to absorb every bit of information about SPS and talk to others. Knowledge, plus wisdom, will give you the determination and confidence to be a better advocate for your health. Do your research. Unfortunately, SPS is not very common, but there are resources available, such as the following listed:

NORD (National Organization for Rare Disorders), a 501(c)(3) organization, is a patient advocacy organization dedicated to individuals with rare diseases and the institutions that serve them. NORD, along with its more than 300 patient organization members, is committed to the identification, treatment, and cure of rare disorders through programs of education, advocacy, research, and patient services. Other sources of information include a website[12] run by the National Library of Medicine National Center for Biotechnology Information.

The United States National Library of Medicine (NLM), operated by the United States federal government, is the world's largest medical library. Located in Bethesda, Maryland, the NLM is an institute within the National Institutes of Health. Its collections include more than seven million books, journals, technical reports, manuscripts, microfilms, photographs, and images on medicine and related sciences, including some of the world's oldest and rarest works.[13]

NINDS (National Institute of Neurological Disorders and Stroke) is part of the National Institutes of Health and is the nation's leading funder of research on the brain and nervous system.[14]

SPSRF (Stiff Person Syndrome Research Foundation) works to raise awareness of Stiff Person Syndrome (SPS), to support research for better treatments and a cure for SPS, while strengthening our community through education and collaboration.[15]

5. Maintain A Healthy Eating Lifestyle

New York City Mayor Eric Adams is an advocate of healthy eating, and his administration recently created new plant-based lifestyle medicine programs throughout the city.[16] He is also encouraging all New Yorkers to join him in plant-based eating, a habit he started after receiving a diabetes diagnosis.

Plant-based nutrition has been shown to protect against the fifteen leading causes of death in the world, including many cancers, and may offer benefits as a disease-modifying tool to improve the management and treatment of these conditions. Results on the effects of plant-based nutrition on breast, prostate, colorectal, and gastrointestinal cancers have been the most extensively studied, and thus have the most published supporting evidence thus far. Whole-food, plant-based diets have been shown to significantly protect against these cancers, as well as additional cancers and other chronic disease states. Nutritional interventions in the prevention of various cancers offer a significant benefit to currently used medical therapies and should be employed more often as an adjunct to first-line medical therapy. Although the effects of diet are becoming more well-known and the role of diet and lifestyle factors in health and disease is gaining more attention and emphasis, the benefits or detriments are still underestimated and undervalued.[17]

A whole-food, plant-based lifestyle is one of the most powerful weapons we have to fight disease, and adopting and maintaining a healthy plant-based diet is essential, and easier than you think for you and your family. I began living a whole-food, plant-based lifestyle about ten years ago and the benefits have been substantial. My risks for heart disease and diabetes have significantly decreased. The choices I make about what to eat are my front-line defense against the progression of SPS. In 2021, I earned the Center for Nutrition Studies' Plant-Based Nutrition Certificate (PBNC) from The T. Colin Campbell Center for Nutrition Studies (CNS).

WEBSITES TO CONSIDER:

The T. Colin Campbell Center for Nutrition Studies (CNS)
https://nutritionstudies.org/about/
Dedicated to promoting the profound effect of food on our well-being, environment, and society, the nonprofit T. Colin Campbell Center for Nutrition Studies (CNS) strives to educate, serve, and advocate for all individuals. By sharing evidence-based knowledge, they aim to inspire and unite individuals to pursue healthier lifestyles, more inclusive communities, and a greener planet.

Ornish Lifestyle Medicine
https://www.ornish.com/
Dean Ornish, M.D., and his colleagues provide plant-based lifestyle medicine, education, and training.

Michael Klaper, MD
https://www.doctorklaper.com
As a physician, consultant, and educator, Dr. Klaper assists individuals in achieving health and wellness.

Milton Mills, MD
https://drmiltonmillsplantbasednation.com
Dr. Milton Mills, a vegan physician, provides medical evidence, education, and research to show that being plant-based/vegan is the best diet for humans.

Eric Adams
https://www.forksoverknives.com/success-stories/eric-adams-new-book-healthy-at-last-soul-food/

Author of Healthy at Last: A Plant-based Approach to Preventing and Reversing Diabetes and Other Chronic Illnesses, Adams's current goal is to bring about change in the healthcare sector by examining the interwoven elements of history, nutrition, and cultural traditions that have had a significant impact on the African American community.

D. Anthony Evans
https://www.hope-theproject.com/d-anthony-evans/
https://www.cheri-inspires.org

D. Anthony Evans has faced and overcome some of life's toughest challenges. Born to a single mother, he was diagnosed with Neurofibromatosis (NF) at birth—a rare condition that causes tumors to grow on nerve tissue. While most are benign, they can become malignant and develop into Malignant Peripheral Nerve Sheath Tumors (MPNST), an aggressive form of cancer. In 2012, D. received the devastating news that he had MPNST. Over eleven months, he underwent nine surgeries, each one posing the risk of paralysis as doctors worked to remove 325 tumors from his body, including one that weighed over two pounds. Given only six months to live, D. refused to give up and fought for his survival. Although the odds were against him, today, he has been able to thrive despite this deadly disease by adopting a plant-based lifestyle.

The Buddhist Chef
https://www.thebuddhistchef.com/recipes/
Healthy, tasty, and planet-friendly vegan recipes.

LEARNING AND DISCUSSION: HOW TO CULTIVATE EMOTIONAL WELLNESS

Nurturing Emotional Wellness:
Dealing with stress is no easy task, especially for those living with a chronic illness. Stress can take its toll and greatly impact one's outlook on life. Prolonged periods of stress can lead to emotions such as frustration, anger, low energy, hopelessness, and even depression, leaving individuals feeling overwhelmed and ready to give up. This not only affects the individual but also their loved ones who are also impacted by the challenges of a chronic health condition.

However, this does not mean that managing stress is impossible. Learning to manage stress is a significant component of controlling our emotions and developing emotional wellness. Often, it's not the situation we experience that fuels our stress but our attitude about the situation. That means you can do more to manage your stress than you may have thought by taking steps to lessen the impact on your body and improve your mental, physical, emotional and spiritual health.

Fortunately, there are numerous scientifically-backed techniques that can help reduce stress levels. These self-help stress management techniques can help ease anxiety and encourage good emotional health. While some may work better than others for each person due to individual differences in facing stressors, it's important to find strategies that are enjoyable and can be practiced consistently. Regular practice is key in effectively managing stress.

What is stress?

Stress is the body's normal and natural biological response to a stressor, which can be positive or negative depending on the situation and the person. It's our reaction to any change we experience in everyday life requiring adjustment or alteration that one must make. The greater the adjustments needed to address the complexities of daily life challenges, the more likely we are to experience stress-induced reactions. For example, you receive tough news about a family member or friend, and your breathing increases, your heart beats faster, and you feel knots in your stomach. If these events are frequent or chronic, your body can become accustomed to responding in this manner, which can harm your body.

Life is full of stressful events such as a relationship ending, financial difficulties, or receiving troubling and unexpected news about your health. Stress events can also be view as positive, like the excitement of the birth of a child, a job promotion, purchasing a new home or retiring and relocating to a bucket list location. A healthy amount of stress, known as eustress, can motivate us to grow and improve in our lives. We need some level of stress to push us towards success and compel us to confront and overcome challenges in our lives. However, too much stress, also known as distress, can be detrimental to our health.

When we experience stress, our brain releases a potent hormone called corticotropin-releasing hormone (CRH), which then prompts the release of other hormones that impact our blood pressure and kidney function. Over time, the impact of stress on hormonal changes in our body can damage our immune system, making us susceptible to infections, heart disease, diabetes, cancer, spasms, pain, anxiety, depression and feelings of hopelessness and doom due to a loss of a spiritual connection and our purpose in life.[23]

While short-term exposure to adapting to change is okay, experiencing constant or long-term adverse events in our life, constant feelings of being under pressure or threatened, or regular exposure to situations we don't feel we can manage or control, eventually, can be unhealthy and damaging to our mind and body.

Additionally, it is more than necessary to acknowledge the unique and concerning challenges faced by Black/African American individuals and families in the United States. The ongoing battle against bigotry, discrimination, prejudice, and racism significantly contributes to the high levels of stress experienced by Black/African American individuals and families. Although everyone faces stressful situations, African Americans are often expected to suppress their anger, leading to a disproportionately high rate of hypertension among them.[24]

As mentioned, occasional stress is not a bad thing. Stress becomes bad stress when it's chronic and ongoing. In these instances, our bodies learn to stay in hyperdrive and does not easily return to a state of balance and calmness. Discovering how to build resilience, proactively avoid stressors, eliminate the root cause of stress, confront and handle stress in a productive manner, and shift your mindset and outlook towards stress are critical components in developing successful techniques for reducing and managing stress.[25] Finding ways to manage this stress is vital to living our healthiest life.

The impact of stress on our spiritual well-being reveals the interconnectedness of our mind, body, and spirit. True wellness is not just about physical and mental health, but also requires attention to our spiritual health. Our best opportunity to achieve optimal health occurs when we prioritize and give equal attention and care to all three aspects of ourselves.

Stress Management Tips

- Get good sleep. Making sure to get enough sleep each night, which is typically at least seven hours for adults, can effectively help manage stress. Getting sufficient quality sleep can also reduce feelings of anxiety, depression, and other mental health problems that are often linked to stress. Here are a few suggestions for achieving better sleep:
  - Set a regular bedtime. Try to be consistent in retiring to bed and waking up at this time daily. To help you to stay consistent, limit daytime naps.
  - Develop a bedtime ritual that helps to prepare your mind and body for sleep. The ritual might include meditating, praying, watching a relaxing television program, listening to soft music, or reading. Some people might also consider taking a hot lavender bath, hot shower, or smudge cardamon, sage, or oregano.
  - Make your bedroom suitable for sleep. A bedroom with a comfortable temperature, dark, and quiet is most helpful. If possible, avoid placing a television or computers in the bedroom. Remember to set the cell phone to do not disturb mode. Use the bedroom only for sleep, intimacy, or sexual activity.
  - Regular exercise is a catalyst for good sleep. Try to exercise during the morning or day, but not before bedtime. Exercising four hours or less before bedtime could make it difficult for your body and mind to transition to fall asleep.

- Avoid eating sweets, caffeinated products, or using nicotine before bedtime. Using these products can impair your ability to sleep.
- If you retire to bed and cannot fall asleep, avoid tossing and turning in bed. Tossing and turning in bed will only make it more difficult for you to fall asleep. Instead, move to a different location and engage in an activity that prepares you for sleep.

If you struggle with falling asleep or experience inconsistent sleep quality, consider using a sleep-tracking device to monitor and document your sleep patterns. Keep track of when you go to bed, how long it takes you to fall asleep, any instances of waking up during the night, what time you wake up in the morning, how rested you feel upon waking up, and your energy levels throughout the day. This information can be shared with your doctor for further review and analysis.

- Should you notice that none of your methods allows you to get good sleep, speak with your healthcare provider for guidance.
- Take time to rest. Taking time to relax and do nothing, even if it's just for a brief period, can have many benefits for both your physical and mental well-being. It can help lower blood pressure, release tension in muscles, and improve mental clarity. On my designated days of doing nothing, I often find myself getting lost in thought and admiring my garden and the wildlife while gazing outside my window or simply closing my eyes and allowing my mind to wander.
- Take a walk. There are many ways to relieve stress that don't require a gym membership. One simple solution is taking a brisk walk for ten to fifteen minutes, which can

quickly release tension from the body. Although any type of walking can be beneficial, maintaining a swift pace may offer even more health benefits. Research has shown that people who walk quickly for about thirty minutes each day have a noticeably lower chance of developing heart disease, cancer, dementia, and mortality compared to those who walk at a slower pace for a shorter amount of time.[26,27] Remember to speak with your doctor before beginning any exercise program.

- Exercise and physical activity can reduce stress. Studies have demonstrated that incorporating exercise and physical activity into one's routine can effectively help manage stress and enhance mental well-being for individuals with chronic illnesses like diabetes, coronary artery disease, and cancer.[28,29]

Engaging in activities such as swimming, brisk walking, cycling, stretching, and Tai Chi for just 30 minutes thrice a week, has been scientifically proven to lower stress levels and help improve your overall quality of life. I have found that practicing Tai Chi and riding my e-bike (electric bicycle) are particularly advantageous for my mental health. After a workout, there is often an immediate sense of improved mood. However, with Stiff-Person Syndrome, exercising can be difficult due to the unpredictable nature of spasms and their varying intensity. There are days when I am unable to complete a workout or engage in light physical activity because of sudden flare-ups. During these moments, I have learned to listen to my body and not push myself. Instead, I take my prescribed medicine allow time to pass, and take advantage of the next opportunity to exercise. My motivation to stay active remains strong, and I make sure to celebrate any progress I make, even if it means not meeting my daily exercise goals on some days.

Even if you don't meet your exercise goals, because you are confronted with limited movement, the value of engaging in physical exercise cannot be overstated. For the 1 billion individuals facing chronic lower limb disability who rely on wheelchairs for mobility, maintaining physical fitness and engaging in regular physical activity for many reasons can be a considerable obstacle and often may feel like it's the norm. Don't give up; it remains crucial to try. Remaining inactive can elevate the risk of developing depression, health complications, and a diminished quality of life. It is impossible to overemphasize the key role of physical exercise in maintaining a healthy lifestyle.[30]

It is advisable to consult with your physician, physical therapist, or other healthcare professionals before starting any exercise or physical activity program. They can help you to determine the best ways for you to include exercise in your daily routine.

- **Eat A Healthy Diet.**

The typical American diet, known as the Standard American Diet (SAD), is composed mainly of animal products, processed foods, and refined carbohydrates. It tends to be high in added sugars, sodium, omega-6 fatty acids, trans fats, cholesterol, and other pro-inflammatory substances that can harm the brain and increase the risk of various physical and mental ailments. Essential nutrients, fiber, and plant-based compounds are often lacking in the SAD. As a result, chronic diseases are the leading cause of death in the US, with the unhealthy SAD being a significant contributing factor.[31,32]

A link between ultra-processed foods, cognitive decline, and impaired brain health has also been established.[33]

Moreover, animal-based products are of particular concern because they contain a pro-inflammatory compound that can aid in producing inflammation in our brain, spinal cord, or nervous tissue that can adversely impact our mental health and lead to depression. According to Dr. T. Colin Campbell, author of The China Study—which is considered one of the most extensive studies on human nutrition in history, conducted through a collaboration between Cornell University, Oxford University, and the Chinese Academy of Preventative Medicine—suggests that controlling the amounts of casein included in our diets can either suppress or promote the growth of cancer cells. Casein is the primary protein found in cow's milk.[34]

Increasingly, scientists are acknowledging that eating animal-based products is causing and contributing to the development of preventable, diet-related sicknesses such as heart disease, diabetes, obesity, and hypertension.

Diet does not just play a role in our physical health but can play a role in mood changes. Sugary processed foods are neurotoxic to the brain and research shows how they can worsen mood, anxiety, and ability to concentrate. Likewise, excessive caffeine, refined sugar, and animal products may lead to heightened feelings of anxiety, encourage addiction, and energy crashes. It is best to avoid these foods to maintain a healthier lifestyle.

But there is hope. By nourishing our bodies with nutritious food and getting enough rest, we are better equipped to handle stress and maintain a balanced state of mind. A diet that includes a variety of fruits, vegetables, whole grains, plant proteins, and healthy fats can provide the necessary nutrients for optimal bodily function and help regulate mood and energy levels while reducing stress.[35]

Additional suggestions for healthy eating choices:

- Ensure that you get the recommended daily servings of fiber. Foods such as apples, bananas, oranges, berries, tomatoes, carrots, and asparagus can help reduce blood cholesterol and blood sugar levels.
- Avoid saturated fats in foods such as bacon, sausage, bologna, ham, butter, milk, and ice cream.
    - Try to eliminate sugars such as corn fructose, maltose, dextrose, sucrose, fructose, glucose, lactose, and polydextrose.
    - Minimize salt use. Foods high in salt and sodium such as potato chips, processed meats, ham, bologna, ketchup, soy sauce, mustard, pickles, or olives can encourage high blood pressure.
    - Reduce alcohol intake. Not only is alcohol devoid of nutrients, but it also packs a high-caloric punch. Alcohol use can also foster the development of high blood pressure, and brain and liver damage, and increase the risk of heart disease.
    - Drink plenty of water daily to prevent dehydration, but not too much. As your doctor what is the right amount of daily water consumption for your specific situation?

Healthy eating habits alone cannot guarantee good health, but they can greatly improve overall well-being and reduce stress-related ailments.

- Emotional or stress eating can be a roadblock to a healthy diet.

  Sometimes, we eat not because we are physically hungry but to fulfill emotional needs or cope with stress. We may turn to food for comfort, to reduce anxiety, to stress relief, to soothe or suppress uncomfortable feelings and situations, or to reward ourselves. This behavior is known as emotional or stress eating, and it is a common practice among many people. These cravings have nothing to do with physical hunger; our bodies do not need nourishment at this time. Rather, it is our chosen reaction to make ourselves feel better in response to a stressful event.

  As an example, yesterday, you learned that you did not get the long-awaited promotion that you worked hard to secure, and on top of that, the check engine light comes on while driving home. Overwhelmed and upset, all you want is to be left alone and comforted. So, without hesitation, you head straight to a restaurant and order your favorite meal - a rack of ribs, red velvet cake, and a bottle of wine. Your appetite knows no bounds as you devour everything quickly without stopping. There are no leftovers in sight. Your stomach is now uncomfortably full, but the satisfaction from indulging in your comfort food brings temporary happiness and contentment.

  Briefly, you felt a sense of childlike joy, recalling memories of your family's celebrations and the delicious meals your mom used to cook. Your dad was unbeatable when it came to ribs, and your aunt's cakes were unmatched. As you devour the ribs and cake, and savor the wine, these memories come back to life, and you can't help but smile with satisfaction. But this feeling is fleeting; it will only last for a few more minutes before reality sets in once again.

When we are faced with stress, perhaps as a way to cope with boredom and loneliness our default response is often to turn to food. Unfortunately, this typically involves reaching for comfort foods from our childhood or younger years, that are sweet, fatty, or high in carbs such as junk food. As we seek contentment, with an "I don't care" attitude, these easily accessible and tempting options may provide temporary relief but are ultimately unhealthy.

Yet, during times of high stress, some people may notice a decrease in their appetite and may either eat less or not eat at all. When asked if they have eaten, they might say things like "I've been swamped with work and just haven't had time to think about food" or "I guess I just forgot." They do not feel hunger cues or have the urge to eat and therefore may end up consuming insufficient nutrients or even skipping meals altogether. This can lead to physical symptoms like headaches, low blood sugar, nausea, significant weight loss, and malnourishment, which can further contribute to feelings of anxiety.

Electing, to choose food in response to a stressful event to soothe our feelings or thoughts won't work. Emotional eating doesn't fix emotional problems. In fact, it usually makes you feel worse. Afterward, not only does the original emotional issue remain, but you may also feel guilty for overindulging, and feelings of distress increase. While you may experience a temporary boost in mood, this momentary comfort comes with the potential price of weight gain and other health complica*tions.*

Strategies To Prevent Emotional Eating:

There are multiple methods for combatting stress eating, and each one is important. However, it's important to recognize and address your specific triggers for emotional eating and control the availability and accessibility of unhealthy foods. These triggers and food choices have a direct impact on exacerbating or causing both physical and mental health issues.

- Know your stressors.

Emotional eating can stem from many stressful events, such as a bad day at work, a fight with a family member or friend, chronic stress, long-term anger, depression, rejection, disappointments, and many other concerns. These might be some of the stressors that spark you to reach for food to comfort yourself. Once you recognize them, you can take steps to avoid them or apply new behaviors to manage the anxiety with something other than food.

- **Purge the Pantry and Refrigerator.**

Clean out your pantry and refrigerator of any sugary treats like candy, cake, or pies. Instead, stock up on fresh or frozen fruits as healthier options. Additionally, eliminate processed foods like chips, deli meats, low-fat yogurt, white bread, canned soup, boxed pasta, and diet snacks from your residence. Replace these with more nutritious choices such as amaranth, barley, brown rice, bulgur, farro, millet, quinoa, sorghum, steel-cut oats, rolled oats, teff, wheat berries, whole wheat products, and wild rice.

- Talk With Your Healthcare Provider.

Suppose you have recognized that you often use food as a source of comfort during times of emotional turmoil and have unsuccessfully tried to find healthier ways to cope, it might be beneficial to seek guidance from your doctor. They can evaluate the situation and determine if consulting with a mental health specialist would be helpful. If therapy is recommended, the counselor can assist you in gaining insight into the specific stressors that trigger your tendency to turn to food for relief.

Food log sheet

For the next thirty days, make sure to copy and keep this log sheet on hand and record everything you consume and how long you exercise. This will allow you to pinpoint potential trouble areas throughout the day and make necessary changes. Pay special attention to moments of stressful eating.

DAYS OF THE WEEK	BREAKFAST	LUNCH	DINNER	SNACKS	EXERCISE	MOOD	STRESSFUL EATING? Y/N
MONDAY							
TUESDAY							
WEDNESDAY							
THURSDAY							
FRIDAY							
SATURDAY							
SUNDAY							
HOLIDAY							

- Learn to Meditate.

  The history of meditation is shrouded in mystery, as the practice has been a part of various cultures and religions for centuries. Although it is difficult to pinpoint its exact origin, some archaeologists estimate that meditation dates back to 5,000 BCE and was prevalent in ancient Egypt as a way of life. Images have been uncovered showing people sitting in familiar postures associated with meditation: cross-legged on the ground, hands resting on their knees, and eyes slightly focused but not fully closed. Texts from Indian scriptures dating back to 3,000 BCE also describe various forms of meditation. These practices eventually spread to China and other countries, becoming an integral part of different societies around the world.[36]

Today, the popularity and use of meditation are increasing as more people discover its many health benefits.

Numerous studies have shown that meditation has positive effects on various health conditions, including:

- Meditation can help to prevent or decrease depression.

  Studies have shown that meditation can have a positive impact on stress which can lead to depression. Stress can trigger the release of cytokines, which are inflammatory chemicals that can affect mood and lead to depression. Research has also indicated that practicing meditation may help reduce levels of these cytokines, further decreasing symptoms of depression.[37,38,39,40]

- Meditation can decrease stress.[41,42,43,44,45,46,47]
- Meditation can improve cardiovascular diseases like hypertension.

  In a series of research studies, it was observed that individuals who consistently engaged in meditation experienced notable improvements in blood pressure, hypertension, heart rate, and cardiovascular diseases.[48,49,50]

- Meditation can protect you from aging-cognitive issues.

There has also been evidence to indicate that meditation not only enhances attention and planning capabilities but may also serve as a safeguard for the brain, effectively protecting against cognitive decline commonly associated with the natural aging process.[51,52,53,54,55,56,57]

- Meditation can boost the immune system.

  Mindfulness mediation appears to be associated with reductions in proinflammatory processes.[58,59,60]
- Meditation can help you manage pain.[61,62]
- Meditation can control anxiety.[63,64,65,66,67]
- Meditation can improve your sleep quality.[68]
- Take time to pray
  - *Prayer therapy and religious/spiritual activities can lessen anxiety and promote hope.*

Aside from other forms of meditation, the positive effects of prayer or prayer therapy on reducing anxiety and promoting optimism in individuals with heart disease have been acknowledged. The role of religion/spirituality in fostering hope for those living with kidney disease has also been confirmed.[69,70,71,72]

Additionally, there is scientific evidence suggesting that engaging in prayer can have beneficial impacts on one's physical well-being. Research studies have demonstrated that individuals who regularly engage in prayer tend to have lower cholesterol levels, experience improved sleep quality, suffer from fewer headaches, and enjoy increased longevity. Notably, those who incorporate prayer or Bible reading into their daily routines are considerably less likely to develop high blood pressure compared to those who do not engage in such activities.[73]

Many individuals turn to prayer as a form of meditation, making it one of the most prevalent and extensively utilized methods. Engaging in prayer and similar practices can yield physical and emotional benefits comparable to other forms of meditation. How one selects how to integrate prayer into one's life is a profoundly personal and intimate pursuit. Whether one chooses to articulate personalized prayers, request intercessory prayers, engage in communal prayer, or recite established prayers, prayer serves as a potent instrument for introspection and forging a connection and conversation with a Source greater than ourselves.

For those affiliated with a religious or spiritual community, seeking guidance from your imam, pastor, priest, rabbi, or spiritual leader on the inclusion of prayer into daily life can be beneficial and perhaps necessary for some. On the other hand, should you not be a member of a religious or spiritual group, or if you are new to praying, you might feel confused or uncertain about how to begin; one option is to think about speaking with an elder in your family or community to get you started.

How to Meditate.

Follow your Breath to Meditate.

Learning to meditate is not very difficult once you understand the importance of proper breathing and how to use your breath. Breathing is the centerpiece and a critical component of meditation and is essential for optimal cognitive and brain functioning, mental capacity, and many other health processes that meditation offers. Our breath provides a powerful means to quiet our thoughts, nourish our bodies, and rejuvenate our spirits.

During my time training in kung fu, qigong, and meditation with the Shaolin Monks and Kungfu Masters from the Shaolin

Temple in China, the importance of using breathing to relax, focus, and find balance was greatly emphasized. At the same time, most people might take their breathing for granted and don't appreciate its value.

A 2016 study revealed evidence providing new insights into the value of breathing and how we can better harness the power of our minds through our breath, suggesting that there may be a clear connection between nasal breathing and our cognitive abilities.[74,75]

Discovering how to meditate requires patience; it takes time to gain control over our thoughts. It may take several sessions before you are able to focus, relax, and find inner peace while noticing your thoughts and feelings without attending to or being distracted by them. In time you will get the feel of meditation and find out how to adapt it to your lifestyle and needs. I do breathing meditation throughout the day, whether I am sitting, lying down, walking, bicycle riding, or practicing tai chi.

Suggested meditation exercise.

- Gently bring your lips together in a closed position. Use your nose to inhale and exhale, for breathing and not the mouth.
- Repeat a phrase silently in your thoughts, or listen to peaceful, melodic music, but refrain from making any sounds or noises. Personally, I like to silently say "I am at peace" or listen to one of these peaceful songs playing in the background:
    - "Ballads" (Coltrane, J). (1963). Ballads {Album} Ballads. Impulse! Records.

- "Can You Stop the Rain" (Grover, W.). (1996). Can You Stop the Rain {Song} on Soulful Strut. Columbia Records.
- "Gethsemane" (Bowman, T.), (Bowman, B). (2021). Gethsemane [Song] on Smooth Vibes, Vol. 1. I.M. Records).
- "Adia" (Elliot, R.). (1999). Adia {Song} on Chill Factor. Blue Note Records.
- "Another Perfect Moment" (Groove, E.), (White, P.). (2016). Another Perfect Moment {Song} on Still Euge. Shanachie Entertainment Corporation.
- "Gospel Truth" (Groove, E). (2009). Gospel Truth {Song} on Sunday Morning. Shanachie
- "You Don't Know Me" (James, B), (Sanborn, D). (1986). You Don't Know Me {Song} on Double Vision. Warner Bros. Records
- "I Know the Plans" (Vail, G). (2002). I Know the Plans {Song} on The Gospel Truth. Greg Vail Music
  - Sometimes, in moments of meditation, when I seek to uncover more about myself and delve into introspection, I listen to a song like "Where Peaceful Waters Flow." (Gladys Knight And The Pips). (1973). Where Peaceful Waters Flow {Song} on Imagination. Buddha Records), or "Marvelous" (Walter Hawkins and The Love Center Choir). (1998). Marvelous {Song} on Love Alive V 25th Anniversary Reunion. Interscope. And as I listen in stillness, I welcome the guidance of my ancestors and embrace inner peace.

- As you slowly inhale through your nose, gently press the tip of your tongue against the roof of your mouth.
- Pause briefly after breathing in.
- As you slowly exhale, relax your tongue in your mouth. Take a moment to pause after each breath. As you focus on your breath, thoughts may arise and try to distract you. Simply observe them without judgment, and then gently guide your attention back to the breath.
- Continue breathing by slowly inhaling and exhaling through your nose for some time. With each exhale, feel the air leave your body gradually. Focus on the sensation of air passing through your nostrils and filling your lungs as you inhale and exhale.

  The length of the pause between inhaling and exhaling varies for each individual. The important thing is that breathing should feel natural and not strained or forced.

After meditating, I usually sit with a glass of water and briefly think about my experience. I often journal or note how my body and mind are at peace, negative thoughts, spasms, and/or pain-free.

Questions to explore about stress management:

Which stress management activities will you be able to incorporate into your everyday lifestyle to help you reduce your stress?

Activities I already participate in include:

____

____

____

____

____

____

____

Activities that I can begin now to help me handle stress in a more productive way include:

____

____

____

____

____

____

____

CHAPTER FIVE

STIFF PERSON SYNDROME AND SEXUAL HEALTH

Physical and emotional intimacy, sexual pleasure, and sexual intercourse in particular are vital to sustaining and adding worth to life. Above all else, sex and intimacy are crucial if you are striving to feel fulfilled when living with a chronic illness. Few experiences can rob you more of feeling like a complete person than being diagnosed with chronic ill health. It can change every aspect of your existence.

To help mediate feelings of distress, sexual activity can be a great source of comfort and pleasure, and help you do your best while living with a never-ending sickness. Reports have found that sex boosts your overall health. Sexual arousal releases chemicals and hormones within the body that act as envoys that help control our body systems and incite a positive mood.[1] Furthermore, sexual activity, precisely intercourse and achieving orgasm, for middle-aged and older individuals could save your life and potentially serve as a powerful defense against the risk of developing heart disease, breast cancer, and prostate cancer. This is refreshing news for many people enduring a major chronic illness.[2] For middle-aged women, a correlation has been found between the quality of partnered sexual activity and various positive outcomes. Women who reported having more fulfilling experiences during intimate moments with their partners also reported an increase in social support, improved emotional well-being, and a heightened awareness of their role in life.[3] Moreover, when confronted with the reality of their expiry, individuals often hold onto the need to engage in sexual activity as a way to affirm their existence. It allows them to feel as if all is well, even when everything else in life has drastically changed.[4]

Additional Health Benefits

Additional health benefits of sexual arousal include:

- The release of feel-good chemicals and hormones that stimulate our reward and pleasure system in the brain – this results in decreased anxiety and supports brain health.
- An easier time sleeping after sex; this is because a natural hormone is released, which promotes feelings of relaxation.
- The promotion of hormone balance, which can help reduce pain. Hormones are released that can help block pain signals.
- A stronger pelvic floor muscles and less urinary incontinence in women who orgasm.[5]

Thinking, talking, or reading about sex when confronted with a chronic illness may be overwhelming and the last thing on your mind, however, it's important to understand that sex and intimacy are essential facets of an individual's quality of life.[6] Throughout my career as a clinician, I have worked with many young and older adults with chronic health issues to understand that the mental, spiritual, and social health characteristics of their sexual life after being diagnosed with a persistent disease are as vital as the carnal facets. The ability to feel good about their body, to have hope, to regain confidence, and to believe that they can establish and continue a sexual life in the wake of their diagnosis is crucial for healthy living. However, it's seldom discussed. It's not over; you don't have to live without a satisfying sex life.

Stiff Person Syndrome and Sexual Dysfunction

Stiff Person Syndrome (SPS) is a chronic illness, and like many chronic illnesses, aspects of the disease and its treatments can harm sexual performance. And while SPS does not impair sexual function, medication, musculoskeletal pain, immobility, fatigue, body image, and spasms can be frustrating and challenging, and negatively affect sexuality, notably since sexual arousal may cause spasms.[7]

Although SPS does not directly impede sexual function, there might be an additional chronic disease onboard that does. Staggeringly, the harsh reality is clear that a significant portion of our society is constantly wrestling with the burden of handling not only one but several chronic diseases, like diabetes, heart disease, and depression. The weight of this reality hangs heavily over the affected individuals and their loved ones as they navigate the challenges and limitations that come with managing multiple health concerns.[8]

What is Sexual Dysfunction?

Sexual dysfunction (SD) is any time displeasure with one's sexual function occurs and causes one to be upset or leads to feelings of unhappiness or distress. It occurs during the sexual response cycle. For men, typical stages of sexual function include arousal, erection, engaging in the sexual act, followed by ejaculation, and a period of rest. Women experience similar stages but with the addition of the possibility of achieving orgasm during the sexual act. However, at any point during these stages, both men and women can encounter the frustrating hurdle of sexual dysfunction. It can arise unexpectedly, interrupting the natural flow of pleasure and connection between partners.[9] In addition, medical illnesses or treatments, physical disability, psychological illnesses and/or treatments, medications, or physical and psychological trauma can all have a detrimental impact on sexual functioning.

Major health conditions including cancer, kidney failure, multiple sclerosis, heart disease, bladder problems, diabetes, heart, and blood vessel (cardiovascular) disease, chronic respiratory illness, lupus, musculoskeletal disorders, human immunodeficiency virus, spina bifida, spinal cord injury, hormonal levels change after giving birth, menopause, as well as low testosterone, can contribute to sexual dysfunction. Chronic illness and sexual problems often go hand in hand.[10] Likewise, medical ailments that produce a decrease in mobility, physical symptoms such as pain, stiffness, and a limited range of motion in hips and knees, fatigue, body image concerns (such as hair loss, joint deformity, rash, scarring, weight change), vaginal dryness and erectile problems are often interrelated with a medical disease(s) and increases the likelihood of developing sexual dysfunction.

Medical treatments such as prostate, breast, testicular, penile, or rectal surgery, radiation, and the following medications are also known to be a factor in promoting sexual dysfunction:

Medicines used to treat high blood pressure and heart conditions, such as:

- Blood pressure medications (e.g., metoprolol, propranolol, chlorthalidone, clonidine)
- Diuretics, including spironolactone, thiazides, and others
- Centrally acting agents, including methyldopa and reserpine
- a-Adrenergic blockers, including prazosin and terazosin
- b-adrenergic (beta) blockers, including propranolol and metoprolol
- Calcium-channel blockers
- Digoxin

Immunosuppressants, like:

- Sirolimus
- Everolimus
- Tacrolimus
- Cyclosporine

Medication used to treat heartburn, stomach ulcers, reflux disease, or other conditions that cause too much stomach acid, including:

- Cimetidine

Medications used to treat cancer, such as:

- Neurotoxic cancer chemotherapies
- Leuprolide (Lupron)
- Goserelin (Zoladex)

Corticosteroids, like:

- Prednisone
- Prednisolone
- Hydrocortisone

Pain Relief Medicines, including:

- Opiates, including synthetic opiates such as Vicodin, OxyContin, and Percocet
- Cannabis (marijuana)

Antiepileptics, such as:

- Dilantin
- Phenytoin
- Primidone
- Valproic acid
- Gabapentin (Neurontin)
- Topiramate (Topamax)

Cholesterol-lowering medications, like:

- Statins and fibrates, or medications used for high cholesterol (e.g., fenofibrate, atorvastatin, simvastatin, fluvastatin, lovastatin, pitavastatin, pravastatin, rosuvastatin)

Psychiatric Medications, including:

- Antidepressants (e.g., escitalopram, sertraline, fluoxetine, venlafaxine)

- Antipsychotics (e.g., aripiprazole, risperidone, paliperidone, haloperidol, thioridazine, thiothixene)
- Benzodiazepines (e.g., lorazepam, clonazepam, diazepam)
- Tricyclic antidepressants, including amitriptyline, doxepin, imipramine, and nortriptyline
- Monoamine oxidase inhibitors (MAOIs), including phenelzine and tranylcypromine
- Anti-mania medications such as lithium carbonate
- Selective serotonin reuptake inhibitors (SSRIs) such as fluoxetine, sertraline, and paroxetine

Hormones, such as:

- Oral contraceptives
- Oestrogens (Estrogens)
- Progesterones

Culturally sanctioned aphrodisiacs, like:

- Cantharidin (Spanish fly)[11]

Recreational Drugs, including:

- Ecstasy
- MDMA
- Tucibi, tuci, tussi or pink cocaine
- Alcohol
- Tobacco
- Hallucinogens

- Narcotics, such as heroin
- Stimulants, such as cocaine and methamphetamines

Sexual dysfunction associated with psychiatric disorders, such as:

- Substance use disorders.
- Past childhood sexual abuse, physical or sexual trauma
- Depression
- Relationship challenges
- Anxiety and stress disorders
- Schizophrenia and schizophrenia spectrum disorders
- Bipolar disorder
- Some over-the-counter antihistamines and decongestants can cause erectile dysfunction or problems with ejaculation.[12]

Prevalence of Sexual Dysfunction

A common issue faced by women is sexual dysfunction, with a significant number reporting struggles with their sexual functioning.[13] The most frequently reported problem is a lack of desire, which appears to be experienced by a considerable portion of women globally. This suggests that many women will encounter some form of sexual dysfunction at least once in their lifetime. Additionally, numerous women may have diagnosable conditions that affect their sexual function.[14] These issues can present as a decrease in desire, difficulties becoming aroused or achieving orgasm, and even discomfort during intimate moments. The frustrating and often distressing condition of sexual dysfunction can have a profound impact on one's well-being and quality of life, leading to feelings of frustration, disappointment, and shame.[15] Among men, the prevalence rates are just as alarming. A staggering majority of men in their middle to older years face challenges with their sexual functioning and erectile dysfunction (ED) is increasingly common with age.[16]

Studies suggest that about 30 million men in the United States are affected by erectile sexual dysfunction.[17] While sexual complications are a common and lingering aftermath of a prolonged disease such as cancer, these impediments are not limited by age or gender, affecting anyone who the disease has touched.[18] As mentioned, problems with sexual functioning, such as desire, arousal, and satisfaction, are a widespread issue that affects many adults in society.[19]

Adult onset of ill health is not a requisite for SD since chronic disease can occur during childhood and adolescence because of congenital disorders. Young people facing these hurdles may experience difficulties establishing, sustaining, or developing relationships and struggle with SD. One significant difference between adults with SD versus children or adolescents is that the latter two usually have no one to discuss their concerns with.

Chronic Illness's Impact on Sexual Functioning

When you are diagnosed with an unremitting health challenge, you might experience nervousness, worries, and trepidations over what the diagnosis means for your life, relationships, self-esteem, and self-worth. Pessimistic thoughts about enjoying sex or physical and emotional intimacy may flood your mind as you search for an answer to the question: what does the future hold for my ability to enjoy a meaningful sexual experience?

Additional concerns you may have:

- Unease about the changes in how your body functions or looks (such as the loss of a breast or testicles) after a medical intervention
- Worry about how your spouse, partner, or sexual companion feels about you
- Feelings of being less attractive, desirable, or confident that you can perform sexually
- Fear that sex may cause pain
- Fretfulness about how your body works or moves
- Apprehension about engaging in physical sexual activity due to a loss of interest (libido/sex drive) or energy

Regrettably, the experience of these anxieties can lead to a deprivation of sex and intimacy. Many couples and individuals are faced with this sequela; it's not uncommon. These marriages and relationships are unhappy and in danger of collapsing. When the marriage fails, it usually results from frustration, loneliness, and rejection towards the chronically ill partner who lacks desire or interest in sex.

Often these individuals bury their minds in the sand and are reluctant to address or talk about the issue. Over time this behavior leads to resentment, and once it emerges, the damage to the relationship can be so unforgiving and severe that resolution can be next to impossible, even with counseling.[20]

Successful self-management of a chronic illness involves many factors, including taking responsibility to recognize symptoms, following medication regimens (take your medicine as prescribed), and keeping your follow-up medical appointments. Without effectively managing chronic illness, your health threats and health screenings will be missed, allowing for troubling consequences of a condition to excel beyond treatment.

Suggestions

Change positions. SPS impacts the musculoskeletal system causing spasms, pain, stiffness, and other problems with movement and function. Hence, you may find that the positions that worked for you before your diagnosis with SPS may no longer be helpful. Being on the top or the bottom may produce significant pain or encourage spasms. Try a side-to-side or spooning position to minimize the onset of pain and spasms; use pillows for support. An adjustable, smart, or waterbed can be extremely helpful. If you are in a wheelchair, consider a model with removable arms.[21]

Make sure you are well-rested before engaging in any activities. A nap beforehand can help enhance your sexual encounter. Try a warm bath. Bathing in warm water before and after sexual activity may keep the muscles loose, relax the joints, and relieve stiffness and pain. Plan sexual activities when pain and stiffness are not present or mild.

Eliminate distractions. Real intimacy means giving each other your full and undivided attention when you have agreed to be together. Put the cell phones in do-not-disturb mode and seek to enjoy the entire presence of each other.

Emotional intimacy is the root of finding your soul mate, and the foundation of all intimate relationships. Try sitting in an intimate space such as by a water view, overlooking the bright lights of a big city, or quietly by the fireplace with your partner and reading a romantic or sexy book to each other.[22]

Keep in mind that the intimacy of sex transcends the physical realm. In a sexual relationship, we come to know more about who we are by unlocking parts of ourselves that may have been hidden, unknown, and that are typically inaccessible while also offering our partner the opportunity to truly see and understand us. It is a kind of dance of trust and vulnerability that binds us together in a unique emotional, physical, and spiritual bond.[23] Emotional intimacy entails learning to share your hearts and not just your bodies.

Try alternatives to intercourse. Many couples learn to expand their sexual repertoire to include oral-genital sex, fantasy, sensory experience, mutual masturbation, and intimate talk. Vibrators, manual stimulation, sex toys, and other intimate acts may also be helpful, especially when sexual activity does not involve a partner.[24] Sensate Focus may also be beneficial. It's an effective exercise developed by Masters and Johnson to resolve sexual difficulties.[25]

Medications to treat SD for some women include Flibanserin (Addyi) and bremelanotide (Vyleesi), the only medications approved to treat hypoactive sexual desire disorder (low sex drive) in women. Hormone therapy is also available depending on your symptoms, and your doctor may recommend topical creams, vaginally administered medications, or hormones taken orally or applied to your skin. If pain is an issue, there are several approaches to reducing pain during intercourse. You can try different sexual positions, vaginal lubricants, or relaxation techniques before sex. You should also speak with your doctor about the use of vaginal dilators.[26]

Medications for erectile dysfunction treatment for many men include Sildenafil (Viagra), Tadalafil (Adcirca, Cialis),

Vardenafil (Levitra, Staxyn), Avanafil (Stendra), Alprostadil self-injection, Alprostadil urethral suppository (Muse), and Testosterone replacement are the available choices. If these medications are ineffective or contraindicated for your situation, try using a penis pump, sometimes called a vacuum pump or vacuum erection device, or consider undergoing a surgical procedure for a penile implant.[27]

Seek professional counseling. Try to find an experienced psychologist who specializes in sexual dysfunction. They will have the expertise and knowledge to help you resolve issues related to sexual dysfunction, even if psychological or physical illness problems foster the SD. In addition, they can collaborate with your medical team and provide you and your spouse or partner with suggestions and additional resources. For particular situations related to SD, you might consider using a sex surrogate or sex doula.[28]

For couples interested in resolving sex complications, researching, and consulting with a certified sex therapist who specializes in tantric techniques may be beneficial. Those who practice tantric sex believe that it can help address issues with sexual dysfunction.[29]

Final thoughts: In contrast, some of these suggestions may not be an option for you, perhaps because of cultural norms, religious beliefs, physical and emotional limitations, preferences, or a decision to maintain absolute celibacy. Whatever decision you make, embrace the journey, and heal with it. And while you are on the road to sexual health, and you possibly encounter others who share their voyage with you, I urge you to respect their decisions. Don't shame or hate them but listen and learn. No one deserves to be treated as a fleeting shadow, almost imperceptible or marked with the scent of invisibility.30 The imperative inference is that chronic illnesses like SPS can cause many changes in your life, however, it doesn't mean you must live without a fulfilling sex life.

LEARNING AND DISCUSSION: SEXUAL INTIMACY AND CHRONIC ILLNESS

Sexual dysfunction: When relationships go wrong

Hints that your relationship was struggling with issues surrounding intimacy and sex through the behavioral signals were sent by your spouse or partner long before they were convinced that the way they are handling their frustration, displeasure, and anger is warranted. A West African proverb from Gambia states, "If your only tool is a hammer, you will see every problem as a nail." In other words, the more limited you are in problem-solving resources, the less likely you are to solve the problem.[31]

These signals can manifest in various ways, from coldness and distance to irritability, avoidance, and violence. It is important to pay attention to these early warning signs and address them before they snowball into feeling that there is no other way to respond except in an escalation of maladaptive, inflexible, and unproductive ways of managing their emotions, resulting in, at the minimum, a verbal eruption.

Warning Behavioral Signals

- Some partners may actually convince themselves that an obliging or composed approach to conflict is good. Pain is seemingly averted, yet it is only compounded as verbal tongue lashings are provoked. However, suppressing their true emotions only makes matters worse when their pent-up frustrations eventually lead to verbal outbursts. This can cause significant damage to the relationship, causing bigger immediate problems and, if not resolved, more significant long-term issues.

- Other spouses or partners, when confronted with an opportunity to express their resentment about the lack of intimacy and sexual activity, might choose to suppress their anger and act as if all is well until one day, there is an angry surge of emotions, and they can no longer pretend that nothing is wrong.
- Yet a few spouses or partners might openly and loudly complain or become verbally and physically aggressive and violent. They want to prove that they are in control of the situation conceivably by snatching up their mate and stripping them of their dignity and self-respect. They might also throw objects around the home and push or hit the person or an object after becoming belligerent. For this, individual domination of their mate's thoughts and emotions solves the problem.
- Still, more than a handful of spouses or partners will respond with a "side-eye" look or react with sarcasm, sighing, pouting, cynicism, and talking down about everything or decisions you are trying to make. Passive aggressively, they will see a problem with everyone, or every thought rendered in an attempt to hurt or play the "get back" game without disclosing or sharing honestly why they are frustrated.

The crippling grip of emotional, sexual frustrations, deprivation, and distress knows no boundaries and can seep into every relationship like a venomous poison. No relationship is immune, but companionships that are hindered by chronic health issues are at a greater risk.

Despite this universal struggle, there are those who choose to deny or hide it. As previously mentioned, refusing to address struggles can lead to malice, heartbreak, and an irreparable relationship despite professional assistance.

However, looking back, there were signs that difficulties with communicating in an empathic, compassionate, yet trustworthy voice had not been practiced, cultivated, or nurtured in these relationships. Nor did the relationships foster fertile soil for a productive conversation to flow. Childish responses to expressing feelings have become ingrained, adopted, and reinforced.

So instead of bottling up your emotions and thoughts, learn to work through them together in a useful and productive manner. It may not be easy, but it is necessary for our emotional well-being and the health of our connections with others.

Moreover, comprehensive management of a chronic health challenge means making and maintaining complex lifestyle changes that involve thinking about sex in new ways. It presents the opportunity to develop creative approaches to initiate sexual activity and practice different ways to be physically, emotionally, and spiritually intimate. You must be willing to explore, for there is more than one way to experience sexual intimacy.

Sexual Intimacy Checklist

What do you believe? After probing the topic of intimacy with a chronic illness, take a moment to reflect on your beliefs and values surrounding this sensitive subject. Read the following statements and carefully consider which ones you believe to hold true and which ones you believe to be false.

1. Sexual intimacy, a beautiful and acrobatic display of passion, involves two vibrant and physically able bodies coming together in an enticing dance.

   TRUE________ FALSE______

2. As my body changes with illness, I am unable to perform as I used to. My body doesn't even move the same way anymore, so why bother trying to be the lover I once was?

   TRUE________ FALSE______

3. Instead of longing for a sexual relationship, I should just be grateful to be alive. It's selfish of me to want to maintain my sexuality.

   TRUE________ FALSE______

4. What good am I? I am worthless if I can't have an organism or reach the same level of pleasure as before.

   TRUE________ FALSE______

5. Will I satisfy my partner? Can they climax with me because of the illness.? These worries plague me, impacting my confidence in bed.

   TRUE________ FALSE______

6. I frequently wonder how I compare sexually to others now that I have an illness.

   TRUE________ FALSE______

7. I have little interest in shopping for clothing, attending events, or being seen in public. I feel ashamed when I look in the mirror, especially if I am undressed.

   TRUE________ FALSE______

8. My doctor has given me the green light to resume my sex life, but I am overwhelmed with fear when I think about being physically intimate again. The idea of causing harm or experiencing pain at the site of my recent surgery terrifies me.

   TRUE________ FALSE______

9. Because of the illness, I worry about getting out of breath or becoming fatigued during sex. The physical activity of sexual intimacy is too much for me to handle.

   TRUE________ FALSE______

10. The physical activity of sex will only worsen the illness or produce a "widowmaker" heart attack.

    TRUE________ FALSE______

What was your response? Did you answer "true" to any of the statements? If every statement was answered with "false", then most likely you do not have distress about engaging in sexual intimacy with a chronic illness.

Or did you answer true to any of the statements, suggesting that you may have fears or concerns about this topic? If so, discussing these with your healthcare provider, who can provide guidance and support, may be helpful. Remember, your feelings and thoughts are valid and deserve to be addressed in a safe and understanding environment.

What is intimacy?

There are countless factors that shape our perception of romantic relationships. From the strength of our community ties, cultural background, and family upbringing, to our own health and how we navigate the constant flow of information in our daily lives. Our experiences, social media influence, peer group, personal beliefs, and place of worship all play a role in how we form and interpret closeness with others.

To truly understand intimacy, it is essential to first define it. While there are many ways to describe this complex concept, at its core, intimacy involves sharing oneself with another person in a way that fosters a deep connection.[32]

It requires baring one's soul—sharing hopes, dreams, fears, humiliations, joys, and sorrows—and being met with acceptance and understanding. It also involves finding a balance between dependence and independence, solitude and togetherness.[33]

As mentioned, our culture and family greatly influence our understanding of intimacy. For example, in Western culture, it is often viewed as the process of sharing emotions, thoughts, experiences, empathy, and support with another person. And in romantic relationships, such as marriage, intimacy is typically built on the concept or feelings of love.[34]

For many people when they hear the word intimacy, they might be tempted to believe that it's all about sex. But, in fact, intimacy involves far more than that.

Types of intimacy

Intimacy is a multifaceted concept, encompassing various types of connections between individuals. Three significant forms of intimacy are physical, emotional, and spiritual. Let's delve deeper into these types of intimacy.

Physical:

Physical intimacy involves being physically close to another person through actions like caressing, cuddling, holding hands, hugging, kissing, and sexual activity. It also encompasses finding attraction in your partner's physical features and making them feel secure through your touch. Here are a few ways you can express your love and desire for your partner through physical touch:

- Gently running your fingers over their skin, teasing and caressing with a feather-light touch to elicit joyful giggles. It's a beautiful moment, watching your partner's eyes light up with happiness. Nothing is more enchanting than seeing them in this state, completely carefree and full of life.
- Let your bodies move freely to the sounds of your favorite music, not worrying about looking silly because this is a moment just for the two of you. This is a playful way to illustrate that you are not afraid of being goofy and that you both can enjoy each other's company.
- As you engage in conversation, gently reach out and make contact with their hand. The warmth of their skin against yours sends a spark through your body, triggering the release of oxytocin - the love hormone. This surge of chemicals floods your brain, making you feel happier and more connected to the person in front of you.[35]

Emotional:

Emotional intimacy requires vulnerability and taking risks by sharing your innermost thoughts and feelings with another person without fear of judgment. Research has shown that human beings must embrace emotional intimacy for healthy development. There are an abundance of ways to express emotional affection towards your partner. Here is an example:

- Your partner listens with compassion and empathy, their reassuring presence lifting some of the weight off your chest. As you release your pent-up frustrations and stresses, they offer words of comfort that soothe and ease your burden. And as you share your emotions, you feel validated, held in a safe haven where you can be vulnerable and heard. In moments of pure happiness, tears of joy may also be shed, further deepening the connection and understanding between you and your confidante. It is in these moments of vulnerability and support that true bonds are formed and strengthened.

Spiritual:

Spiritual intimacy involves sharing one's beliefs and connecting on a deeper level with another person. This does not mean having the same beliefs but instead being open to each other's ideas about life's purpose and connection to a higher power. It can create a sense of closeness and allow for envisioning a shared future together.

Here are a few ways you can deepen your bond with your partner through spiritual intimacy:

- Incorporating shared spiritual practices into your relationship, such as sitting in silent meditation, fervent prayer, or attending sacred religious services, can be an incredibly powerful way to strengthen and enrich your spiritual connection. By engaging in these activities together, you open yourselves up to a deeper level of understanding and intimacy, creating a sacred bond that transcends the physical realm. As you join your hearts and minds in these moments of contemplation and worship, you will feel a sense of oneness with each other. These shared experiences will not only deepen your spiritual connection but also bring you closer together as partners.

Let's review

In summary, intimacy is a feeling of trust and comfort that is established between two people. It can occur in different types of relationships, not just romantic or sexual ones, and is essential for building strong and meaningful connections based on vulnerability and closeness.

Developing intimacy requires effort and dedication, but by cultivating these different types of intimacy, you can improve your relationships and have a positive impact on your mental, physical, and spiritual well-being.

Intimacy in modernity

It is worth noting that attitudes and behaviors towards intimacy vary greatly across cultures and time periods, and society's views on love have evolved.[36]

Exercise: Do you frequently experience frustration with intimacy?

True________ **False**______

Take a moment to observe the *Fear of Intimacy Scale* below. The one on the left is for your level of intimacy, while the one on the right represents your spouse or partner's level. For each type of intimacy, rate yourself accordingly. If you believe that you excel in demonstrating this type of intimacy, give yourself a rating of 10. However, if you feel that you do not demonstrate intimacy in this area, give yourself a 1. It is important to note that it is possible that you demonstrate healthy behaviors a little within each category, so your rating may fall somewhere between 1-10. Use the same scale of measurement for your spouse or partner as well.

Once both of you have finished the exercise, share your findings and use them as a basis for discussing intimacy with one another. Here are some potential conversation questions to help guide your discussion.

- What do you view as each other's greatest obstacle when it comes to intimacy, and what is the reasoning behind it?
- Can you provide any personal examples or experiences that influenced your answer?
- What is legitimate about how you feel about intimacy?
- What is legitimate about how your spouse or partner feels about intimacy?
- How does the management of how you both address intimacy leave you both feeling trapped, angered, or disappointed?
- If we now have a better understanding of each other's concerns or fears surrounding intimacy, how can we approach it in a more meaningful way?
- How can this knowledge help us improve our shared experiences of intimacy?

FEAR OF INTIMACY RATING SCALE

PHYSICAL INTIMACY		
Questions	**Your Answers**	**Spouse/Partner Answers**
I prefer no physical contact.	① ② ③ ④ ⑤ ⑥ ⑦ ⑧ ⑨ ⑩	① ② ③ ④ ⑤ ⑥ ⑦ ⑧ ⑨ ⑩
I am open to hugs and hand-holding	① ② ③ ④ ⑤ ⑥ ⑦ ⑧ ⑨ ⑩	① ② ③ ④ ⑤ ⑥ ⑦ ⑧ ⑨ ⑩
I am open to cuddling.	① ② ③ ④ ⑤ ⑥ ⑦ ⑧ ⑨ ⑩	① ② ③ ④ ⑤ ⑥ ⑦ ⑧ ⑨ ⑩
I am open to kissing.	① ② ③ ④ ⑤ ⑥ ⑦ ⑧ ⑨ ⑩	① ② ③ ④ ⑤ ⑥ ⑦ ⑧ ⑨ ⑩
I am open to having sexual intercourse.	① ② ③ ④ ⑤ ⑥ ⑦ ⑧ ⑨ ⑩	① ② ③ ④ ⑤ ⑥ ⑦ ⑧ ⑨ ⑩

EMOTIONAL INTIMACY		
Questions	**Your Answers**	**Spouse/Partner Answers**
I am emotionally connected.	① ② ③ ④ ⑤ ⑥ ⑦ ⑧ ⑨ ⑩	① ② ③ ④ ⑤ ⑥ ⑦ ⑧ ⑨ ⑩
I listen with compassion and empathy.	① ② ③ ④ ⑤ ⑥ ⑦ ⑧ ⑨ ⑩	① ② ③ ④ ⑤ ⑥ ⑦ ⑧ ⑨ ⑩

I offer words of comfort.	① ② ③ ④ ⑤ ⑥ ⑦ ⑧ ⑨ ⑩	① ② ③ ④ ⑤ ⑥ ⑦ ⑧ ⑨ ⑩
I am willing to share my inner-most thoughts and feelings.	① ② ③ ④ ⑤ ⑥ ⑦ ⑧ ⑨ ⑩	① ② ③ ④ ⑤ ⑥ ⑦ ⑧ ⑨ ⑩
I provide a safe haven and a deep emotional bond.	① ② ③ ④ ⑤ ⑥ ⑦ ⑧ ⑨ ⑩	① ② ③ ④ ⑤ ⑥ ⑦ ⑧ ⑨ ⑩

SPIRITUAL INTIMACY

Questions	Your Answers	Spouse/Partner Answers
I am open to praying or meditating together.	① ② ③ ④ ⑤ ⑥ ⑦ ⑧ ⑨ ⑩	① ② ③ ④ ⑤ ⑥ ⑦ ⑧ ⑨ ⑩
I share my beliefs about God or spiritual enlightenment.	① ② ③ ④ ⑤ ⑥ ⑦ ⑧ ⑨ ⑩	① ② ③ ④ ⑤ ⑥ ⑦ ⑧ ⑨ ⑩
I am open to praying or meditating together.	① ② ③ ④ ⑤ ⑥ ⑦ ⑧ ⑨ ⑩	① ② ③ ④ ⑤ ⑥ ⑦ ⑧ ⑨ ⑩
I am open to exploring a deeper level of understanding one another.	① ② ③ ④ ⑤ ⑥ ⑦ ⑧ ⑨ ⑩	① ② ③ ④ ⑤ ⑥ ⑦ ⑧ ⑨ ⑩
I feel close to you when we're in worship together.	① ② ③ ④ ⑤ ⑥ ⑦ ⑧ ⑨ ⑩	① ② ③ ④ ⑤ ⑥ ⑦ ⑧ ⑨ ⑩

CHAPTER SIX

ON LAUGHTER

I was first introduced to the benefit of laughter during graduate school in the early 1980s. I was working on my doctorate in clinical psychology when the work of Norman Cousins and Bernie Siegel was mentioned. In Cousin's book, *Anatomy of an Illness as Perceived by the Patient,* he describes how his symptoms of ankylosing spondylitis improved using humor. Reportedly, he watched comedy films, including the Marx Brothers and Candid Camera. Cousins discovered a strange realization that a few minutes of deep, belly-aching laughter miraculously affected his body. It was a powerful antidote that brought him moments of joy amidst the trial of pain. And even after the laughter subsided and his pain returned, he would switch on the film again, leading to another period of relief. It was a simple remedy, but one that brought immeasurable relief.[1]

In his book, *Love, Medicine and Miracles,* Dr. Bernie Siegel emphasizes the importance of finding time throughout the day to experience spontaneous laughter while maintaining a child-like sense of humor. For Dr. Siegel, laughter is like a magical elixir that can transform our body chemistry and flood us with youthfulness and vitality. It has the power to mend even the deepest wounds. It has the power to transform relationships and bring people closer together. And when we cry, whether from joy or sorrow, we wash away the toxins that have built up within us.[2]

Since their work, the interest in laughter as a potential therapeutic agent has evolved in society and medical literature.

Physiological Benefits of Laughter

- Laughter brings more oxygen to your blood and increases your heart rate. This benefit helps to decrease the risk of a heart attack.[3]
- When you laugh, at least three hormones are activated: dopamine, endorphins, and serotonin. These hormones are known as the body's feel-good chemicals. When these hormones are released, they notify your body that all is well and that you are happy and in a good mood. Additionally, when these hormones are released, they trigger the body's natural healing process and ease pain symptoms.[4]
- Laughter can help to relax your muscles, improve blood circulation, and ease your ability to breathe. Improving blood circulation can also help to decrease the opportunities of suffering from cardiovascular diseases.[5]
- Each time you laugh, about 400 muscles are involved. So, laughing makes our muscles stronger and well-shaped.
- Laughter has been identified as an essential agent in decreasing inflammation. While the exact mechanism of action is unknown, researchers found that rheumatoid arthritis patients who laughed after listening to the comic story had increased levels of anti-inflammatory chemicals in their blood.[5]

- Laughter decreases physical pain receptors.
- Laughter reduces cellular decay.[6]
- Laughter lowers blood sugar levels.[7]

Psychological Benefits of Laughter:

- The release of endorphins, dopamine, and serotonin (feel-good) chemicals decreases physical and mental pain. If you are feeling sadness, grief, unhappiness, or experiencing negative emotions or depression, try flooding your brain with the release of these hormones by routinely laughing. Laughter will help to alleviate these symptoms.
- Laughter is a key to a good night's sleep.[8]
- Laughter diminishes anxiety and the impact of trauma.[9]
- Simon Wiesenthal, a survivor of the Nazi death camps, who dedicated his life to documenting the crimes of the Holocaust and to hunting down the perpetrators still at large, seems to believe that humor is an armored shield for the oppressed against the pain and suffering they endure every day. It allows them to fight back and find hope and strength in dire circumstances.[10]
- Laughter increases your odds of survival and longevity.[11]
- Laughter improves self-esteem and mood in cancer patients.[12]
- Laughter has positive effects on bronchial asthma.[13]
- Laughter is beneficial in people with severe chronic obstructive lung disease.[14]
- Laughter improves cognitive abilities in older adults.[15]
- Laughter and its effects on Parkinson's Disease.[16]

- Laughter has a positive impact on people with Schizophrenia.[17]

Around the same time, I was introduced to the work of Norman Cousins and Bernie Siegal, M.D., and my wife, and I attended a comedy show at the local community college. We were seated close to the stage and positioned in the center of the row. The auditorium was sold out. I will never forget that night. He made us laugh so hard, that we were literally on the auditorium floor. We were gasping for air, and our cheeks, belly, and face were sore. We looked at one another and laughed harder. I looked up, seemingly making eye contact with him, and begged him to stop. However, he had us and would not let go. He had us trapped, and I believe that he knew it. My side ached, and I thought I would pass out. That night, I laughed like the Egyptian god, Geb.

A Laugh Buddy is a Must-Have

There's something special about sharing a laugh with a friend than laughing alone. The power of laughter seems amplified tenfold when enjoyed in the company of another person. The exchange of laughter between two people often creates an unbreakable bond.[18]

A laughing buddy can allow you to feel unrestrained joy. Sharing a laugh with a buddy can help alleviate your worst fears, your deepest aches, and moments of depression or sadness. A laugh buddy can also help you to recover from the experience of trauma, grief, and hardship. It's important to find someone to check in with you to make sure you spend time laughing throughout the day. It's no secret that laughing with others brings us closer together, creates a deep sense of camaraderie, and strengthens social connections that have positively impacted many aspects of our health.[19] Having a laughing buddy is a force.

About twenty years ago, I met a friend, colleague, and mentor who may have been one of the happiest people I've ever met. Dr. S. was of the Jewish faith. Her humor was a mixture of Groucho Marx, Phyllis Diller, Joan Rivers, Richard Pryor, and Dave Chapelle. Her humor was cutting-edge and seemingly, straight out of Comedy Central. Dr. S. was great at slipping in jokes during some of the most intense situations and interactions. Our clinical job was stressful, but she was a smile seeker and brought healing to my mind during the heavy times.

In 2013, I received a phone call from Dr. S. We were no longer working at the same facility, and our interaction had waned over the years. But the precious memories of our social interactions remained close to my heart. Dr. S. asked if we could meet for lunch. I noticed during the phone call that her quick wit was toned down, and I knew something was wrong.

We met for lunch, and she revealed she had stage four breast cancer. It was very tough news to digest. I hugged her and assured her she had my support as she cried. I asked how I could best support her, and she asked if we could be laugh buddies. I eagerly agreed.

So, weekly, we exchanged jokes via email and text for the next seven years. According to humor expert Allen Klein, "Have a humor buddy you can do humor emailing with."[20] Yes, some jokes were raw, born out of pain, but extremely funny. After all, she was a mixture of some of the most incredible standup comics to have lived. We enjoyed the same type of humor.

Sharing humor when things seem dreary helped prevent her from giving up and sinking deep into depression. While sad moments and asking the "why" question are understandable, you must be careful not to give up on hope. Dr. S. often mentioned that the moments spent exchanging jokes strengthened her resolve. Laughing with a buddy provided comfort and assured her that she was not alone. It also enhanced our relationship. Dr. S. made her transition in 2020 surrounded by her family.

Having a laugh buddy can help you:

- Develop a positive frame of mind. Coming face to face with hardship should not be considered flawed. What is important is how we deal with it. Laughing with a buddy can take the focus away from negative thinking, encouraging you to feel more cheerful.
- Change your perspective. When life throws curve balls, and we feel scared, confused, and overwhelmed, we can become consumed with the challenge and lose hope. This is when having someone to laugh with can help us pause and find the support to move forward. Getting stuck in the problems is not helpful. But denying the reality of the situation is not optimal either. Humor has the power to shift our perspective and encourage us to see challenges as opportunities rather than threats.[21] Its infectious nature can quickly spread, uplifting those around us.[22]

A laugh buddy has social benefits. Laughing with someone creates a collective bond and prevents us from facing tragedies alone.[23] A laugh buddy can help you bring more laughter into your life; there is now laughter for two.

Finding a laughing buddy is not always an easy task. This is true, especially if we are confronted with an illness that makes us uncomfortable. Our physical appearance and lifestyle interruptions, or the use of observable medical devices, may make us feel ashamed because we believe that everyone is looking. We may be less motivated to find time to laugh or to look for someone to laugh with. This can catalyze social isolation, depression, and disease escalation. There is nothing healthier than bonding with people through the relationship of a laughing buddy.

Additionally, it can be challenging to find a laughing buddy if the attempts to share humor are misunderstood by a laugh buddy's spouse, family member, or others. Not everyone shares the same humor, nor are they aware of the benefits of sharing laughter. A spouse may become jealous of the relationship and be offended if they "ear-hustle" or message snoop the conversation. The situation can become embarrassing. Not everyone can handle a joke. However, the gamble is worth it, so go for it.

Finding someone you connect with and have fun with is vital in growing through health challenges. It helps if the person shares your outlook on life. Bonding together will allow you to develop a special relationship that has meaning within the soul of both of you.

How Do I Find Ways To Laugh More?

If you are searching for ways to help yourself to laugh more, there are several things you can do. Here are a few strategies that I have found helpful to encourage me to laugh daily:

- Set time aside each day to laugh, even if I don't feel like it. Once I start watching a funny movie or listening to a humorous story, I soon laugh, and feelings of happiness begin to surface. The first step to happiness is to seek it even if you don't feel like it.
- Keep a humor resource space. In this space, add your favorite funny movies, podcasts, books, jokes, stories, or anything you find funny. So, if you are feeling down

or noticed that you haven't laughed in a while, use your resources. You don't have to think about searching for humor, you have it tucked away.

- Engage with friends. We are socialized to laugh more in a group. It can feel very refreshing to talk to someone and experience laughter through a stream of interactions and conversations. Therefore, make sure you spend time with friends who make you laugh regularly. Find those people you can be yourself with unconditionally and allow them to see who you are through laughter.
- Laugh at yourself. One of the best features of Dr. S. was not that she could make you laugh under stressful situations, but that she could poke fun at herself. While she was intellectually sophisticated and intelligent, she also revealed that she was in touch with humanity. She was human and had vulnerabilities, just like all. Life is all about how you approach things. So even if you're going through hard times, look for the good or the humor. This will positively impact your outlook, health, and overall quality of life.

There is nothing humorous about living with, growing through, and learning to thrive with Stiff Person Syndrome. However, finding ways to experience fun through laughter helps me make it through the day and night. My nighttime can be very challenging. Laughing takes the stress off the dreaded moments of spasms and incapacitation. I strongly encourage the use of daily laughing. The benefits of laughing will vary by person, but you will see yourself progressing in your ability to handle stressful self-doubting moments, and your outlook on coping with the disease will improve.

Laughter is the Best Medicine: My Favorite Remedies

"There's something off-putting about a person with a stern, unyielding expression."

—*Maya Angelou (1998)*

"A good laugh is like a burst of sunlight streaming through a window, illuminating every corner of the room with warmth and brightness."

—*William Thackeray (1851)*

"When we can laugh at something, it becomes easier to handle and overcome."

—*Joan Rivers (2010)*

"There is no need for outdoor exercising, just share laughter among friends."

—*Norman Cousin (2016)*

"The corners of a genuine smile turn upwards transform the whole face with warmth and bring joy to those who need and see it."

—*Phyllis Diller (Date Unknown)*

"Not many people can laugh and make love at the same time. But truly, the source of their love and laughter is one and the same, a place that not many have the privilege to visit."

—*James Baldwin (1974)*

"Laughter brings two souls closer together with each heartfelt chuckle."

—*Victor Borge (Date Unknown)*

"Laughter that brings a sense of release is echoed from the painful empty spaces of the heart."

—Groucho Marx (1960)

"A gentle reminder to let go and surrender to the uncontrollable laughter."

—Osayi Osar-Emokpae (2011)

"Revel in joy and humor and seize every opportunity to laugh."

—Will Rodgers (Date Unknown)

"There are times when laughter is the best medicine for your soul."

—Veronica Roth (2014)

"God looked down with a smile when you genuinely rejoice and laugh from the depths of your heart."

—Martin Luther King, Jr. (Date Unknown)

"I can't help but have a soft spot for those who can make me laugh. I honestly believe that being able to make someone laugh is one of the most valuable qualities a person can possess."

—Audrey Hepburn's quote from the book How to be Lovely by Melissa Hellstern (2005)

"Humor can have a cleansing effect on our minds and spirits, leaving us feeling rejuvenated and revitalized."

—Langston Hughes (2002)

"I struggle to find a common factor among those I admire or hold in high regard, yet among those I love, there is one: they all can make me laugh."

—W. H. Auden (1963)

"The one remedy that money can't buy from a store is laughter."

—Michael Bassey Johnson (June 4, 2016)

"Throughout humanity, there have been two things that we have consistently shared: animosity and amusement. I take pride in using humor as a means to diminish hatred."

—Richard Pryor (2004)

"I live by this motto: find joy in life and seek out happiness instead of dwelling on sadness. Laughter has been my lifesaver in times of unhappiness."

—Red Skelton (Date Unknown)

"As I step onto the stage, I prepare to deliver a performance that will ease your mind and alleviate your daily burdens."

—Bernie Mac (Date Unknown)

Laughter is typically a joyful experience, promoting happiness and connecting us with others. Yet, in certain situations, excessive or intense laughter can result in temporary discomfort that manifests as spasms. It is essential to balance our enjoyment of laughter with awareness of our physical limits to avoid unintended consequences.

LEARNING AND DISCUSSION: HOW TO ENJOY THE BENEFITS OF LAUGHTER

You don't have to wait for something funny to happen to experience laughter. There are ways to cultivate a sense of joy and playfulness in your daily life, even when you're going through difficult times. Consider these tips and techniques for incorporating more humor into your life, regardless of the challenges you may be facing.

Laughing with others:

- When did you last spend time with people who make you laugh?
  - Besides the laughter, what did you enjoy most about your time together?
  - If possible, how can you spend more time with them?

What makes you laugh?

- When did you last watch a funny movie, TV show, podcast, or social media video?
- Have you ever laughed so hard that tears streamed down your face, barely able to breathe, or clutched your side with the exertion? Can you describe what made you laugh?

Keep A Laugh Diary:

Keep a laugh diary over the next thirty days and record each time you experience a "good laugh." Examples of a "good laugh" can be described as laughing with family or friends at a joke (a communal time of sharing joy), letting loose while spontaneously laughing with chuckles, snorts, and grunts, doubling, or bending over with "face stretching" laughter, holding on to one's stomach in a humorous minute of uninhibited amusement, or covering their mouth in a split second of surprised delight before spurting out a drink because of your laughing outburst. Record the following information, and at the end of thirty days, explore how laughter eased your stress and pain.

- Laughter uplifted my mood. YES NO
- Laughter eased my earlier tension. YES NO

Can you list five funny movies, TV shows, podcasts, or social media videos that made you laugh?

1. ______________________________
2. ______________________________
3. ______________________________
4. ______________________________
5. ______________________________

Five Activities To Do For A Laugh.

1. Bring something that appears delicious and has an excellent presentation but actually has a horrible taste to a potluck get-together and watch people as they take a mouthful or a bite. Examples: donut burger, Asparagus water, or fairy bread.[24]
2. Sit at a park or outdoors at a restaurant, and people watch; you will most definitely see something or someone that will make you laugh.
3. Join a laughter yoga group. Laughter yoga, or *hasyayoga*, is a deliberate practice involving physical movement

and specialized breathing techniques to induce prolonged laughter.[25]

4. Get a subscription to the comics to read and laugh daily.[26]
5. Visit Gagster at https://gagstergifts.com/ for additional suggestions and prepare for a barrage of funny expletives, shouts, screams, and a string of exclamations resembling *Saturday Night Live* satire or comedy performance.[27]

CHAPTER SEVEN

FINAL THOUGHTS

"There is a force within each of us that shines brighter than any darkness, a power that can never be taken away, a light that guides us through even the toughest of times."

—*Tracy Scott, Psy.D.*

Over the last six months of shaping and pruning a couple of years of research into this book, I've revisited Dr. Daniel Black's work, paraphrased one of his essential concepts, and listened to the program from which it originates fifty or more times.[1] And honestly, I often review the selection in deep thought, understanding that the challenge of overcoming adversity can be a journey of pain, revelation, discovery, and healing. I don't know where you are in your healing adventure. I had never imagined I would be at this point, but here I am. Each time I am confronted with the challenge of thriving through adversity, I try to remember at least one crucial concept: The Creator does have a plan and purpose for each of us. And no matter the distress I endure, it can never be more critical than understanding that my life has meaning and a purpose.

When finding out that you have been diagnosed with a disease, illness, or syndrome that is chronic or life-threatening, you may feel discouraged and afraid of the voyage ahead. It may be easy to understand why during times of distress, many people question whether their life has a purpose; and if so, what?

You went shopping, fishing, or ate your favorite meal to feel better. People often turn to alcohol, drugs, sex, gambling, and sports, disengage physically and emotionally, withdraw from social activities, act aggressively, or become workaholics trying to find relief.

Some may deal with stressful situations by hurting themselves, such as cutting, scratching, picking at scabs or wounds, or refusing to be responsible for their healthcare. Unfortunately, a few will attempt or commit suicide.

These behaviors are directed at coping with the dreadful news of an illness. They may bring immediate pleasure and gratification. They can make you feel better and take the edge off. But, you find out that it does not last. You recognize that you have exalted yourself, and the maladjustment of coping did not give you the fulfillment you sought. You still feel overwhelmed, anxious, and awful, yet you may still believe that the meaning of life must be wrapped in pleasure.

At this point, many people begin to accept that they cannot control their lives, and they conceive that there is no hope; they conclude their outcome is unchangeable and assume they are helpless, no matter what they do. This inclination also causes stress and leads to despair, depression, and giving up. It starts in the mind with pessimistic thoughts and ends with ultimately questioning the purpose of life.

The answer is yes; there is a purpose for your life and incumbrance we all must carry; finding that purpose is the foundational key to overcoming and thriving through adversity.

I trust that as you understand this concept, it will help you find comfort in your journey and help you know the answer to the question, "Why me?" Concentrate on finding your agency and less on the trauma. The revelation you will discover is not so you can keep it to yourself but, more importantly, so that you can provide the same measure of comfort, empathy, and compassion to others.

I hope this book leads you to this discovery; perhaps it will make it much easier for you to stay healthy while living with SPS. I invite you to use it as a reference tool to keep on a striving and thriving course consistently.

The key is to recognize that life has meaning and a purpose. Life rarely goes as expected.

How am I doing?

These days....

SPS encourages me to sit quietly in silence, look back over my life, and visualize the bodily changes and the memories of remembering when I could...back then I had no idea what was in store. Perchance that was a good thing.

SPS encourages me to vigilantly listen for information or media accounts of new treatment options and patients' stories of SPS or stories of hope while living with a chronic illness. I find myself rooting for those stricken with a lifelong illness or disease to live their best life despite the impact that the sickness has on their physical body, mind, and spirit. I sometimes catch myself watching programs or listening to podcasts that would be a no-no ten years ago. How funny and amazing is this?

SPS encourages me to have occasions of sadness, especially when the spasms will not allow me to rest or sleep. My lift chair holds many of my private heartbeat moments of moaning painful expressions and wondering what lies ahead. If it could only talk back-would you believe me if I told you that it does… just kidding.

SPS encourages me to cry sometimes as my body aches, and I must increase the dose of the medication to feel relief. For a minute, I think, why me…then I answer, SPS, let's dance…I am built for this.

SPS encourages me to acknowledge the scar tissue throughout my body, the remnants of spasms. I walk like I am drunk, and a couple of times, while out on a walk, the police asked if I needed help. I replied thanks but it's Stiff-Person Syndrome. Do you want to smell my breath?

SPS encourages me to say no to toxic people and relationships. Your world of companions shrinks with SPS but friendship with narcissists is not advisable.

Since my diagnosis, seven years ago, I have taken every step to corral my illness into a manageable state. I have implemented all the ways mentioned in this book, from a healthy eating lifestyle to meditation and tai chi, and all in between to ensure that I continue to make sure my agency is greater than the trauma of SPS. So far…so very good. But don't be fooled; thriving with SPS is a daily battle, and unfortunately, the war never ends. SPS, may I have this dance?

NOTES & REFERENCES

Preface

1. https://www.bbc.com/news/entertainment-arts-63904242; https://www.theguardian.com/music/2022/dec/08/celine-dion-diagnosis-rare-neurological-disorder-Stiff Person-syndrome

Chapter 1: Mystery Illness

1. Vidor, K., Fleming, V., Cukor, G., Thorpe, R., Taurog, N., & LeRoy, M. (1939). The Wizard of Oz. Metro-Goldwyn-Mayer (MGM), or the robot from The Twilight Zone; (Episode 5.8 "Uncle Simon" Original air date: November 15, 1963, Writer: Rod Serling Director: Don Siegel.
2. https://dailymed.nlm.nih.gov/dailymed/lookup.cfm?setid=5648c772-50cb-4961-996e-e68a8eb699ea
3. https://www.ncbi.nlm.nih.gov/pmc/articles/PMC1480257/
4. Sperry, L. (2006). *Psychological treatment of chronic illness: The biopsychosocial therapy approach.* American Psychological Association.
5. Kyverna's KYV-101 receives U.S. FDA RMAT designation for KYV-101 in treating patients with Refractory Stiff-Person Syndrome | Kyverna Therapeutics. (n.d.). Kyverna Therapeutics. See https://ir.kyvernatx.com/news-releases/news-release-details/kyvernas-kyv-101-receives-us-fda-rmat-designation-kyv-101). (Mph, I. C. (2024, August 5). FDA grants Regenerative Medicine Advanced Therapy designation to Kyverna's KYV-101 for Refractory Stiff-Person Syndrome. Neurology Live. https://www.neurologylive.com/view/fda-grants-regenerative-medicine-advanced-therapy-designation-kyverna-kyv-101-refractory-sps)

6. https://my.clevelandclinic.org/health/articles/9288-chronic-illness-and-depression
7. Cassell EJ. The nature of suffering and the goals of medicine. New York: Oxford University Press, 1991.
8. https://www.cdc.gov/chronicdisease/index.htm
9. https://my.clevelandclinic.org/health/articles/4062-chronic-illness
10. https://www.cdc.gov/chronicdisease/index.htm
11. https://adaa.org/understanding-anxiety/chronic-illness-disease-anxiety-depression
12. Muzzin LJ, Anderson NJ, Figueredo AT, Gudelis SO. The experience of cancer. Soc Sci Med. 1994;38:1201–1208. 10.1016/0277-9536(94)90185-6
13. 1692, Fables of Aesop and Other Eminent Mythologists with Morals and Reflections by Sir Roger L'Estrange, Abstemius's Fables, Fable CCCXIII, Quote Page 274 and 275, Printed for R. Sare, T. Sawbridge, B. Took, M. Gillyflower, A. & J. Churchill, and J. Hindmarsh, London

Chapter 2: The Impact of Living with an Invisible Illness

1. Vickers, Margaret H. (1998). "Life at Work with "Invisible" Chronic Illness (ICI): A Passage of Trauma - Turbulent, Random, Poignant." Administrative Theory & Praxis. 20 (2): 196–210. ISSN 1084-1806
2. https://www.verywellmind.com/what-is-invisible-illness-you-dont-look-sick-5119873
3. https://stiffperson.org/?submissionGuid=8ecc3fc1-1e71-428a-a316-c1ef82443207
4. https://www.hopkinsmedicine.org/health/wellness-and-prevention/forgiveness-your-health-depends-on-it
5. https://understandingmyositis.org/invisible-illness
6. https://www.yalemedicine.org/conditions/Stiff Person-syndrome
7. https://pubmed.ncbi.nlm.nih.gov/24995360
8. Oxford University Press; American First Edition, July 31, 2013.

9. https://robertroybritt.medium.com/why-is-empathy-so-hard-8eb08e70478d
10. https://psycnet.apa.org/doiLanding?doi=10.1037%2Fxge0001073
11. https://www.researchgate.net/publication/256487303_SOCIAL_NETWORKS_AND_SOCIAL_SUPPORT_AS_DETERMINANTS_OF_HEALTH)
12. https://www.ncbi.nlm.nih.gov/pmc/articles/PMC3017348
13. Goleman, Daniel. *Emotional Intelligence: Why It Can Matter More Than IQ*. 2006
14. Albert Bandura, Social Learning Theory. 1977 Englewood Cliffs, N.J.: Prentice Hall
15. https://www.ncbi.nlm.nih.gov/pmc/articles/PMC5513638
16. https://www.sciencedaily.com/releases/2018/03/180312085124.htm
17. Scott, 2010
18. https://bgcc.org/dr-martin-luther-king-jr-club/, Sears YMCA https://www.realskatestories.com/ymca-chicago-skating
19. http://marillacstvincent.org/history/marillacsocialcenterhistory/asharedstorymarillacsocialcenterandeastgarfieldpark.html
20. https://www.huffpost.com/entry/lessons-of-compassion-fro_b_7868940
21. https://www.sciencedirect.com/science/article/abs/pii/S0191886919306567
22. https://repositorio.umaia.pt/bitstream/10400.24/1580/1/Immature_Personality_.pdf
23. Baires, N.A., Catrone, R. & May, B.K. On the Importance of Listening and Intercultural Communication for Actions against Racism. Behav Analysis Practice 15, 1042–1049 (2022). https://doi.org/10.1007/s40617-021-00629-w

Chapter 3: Turning to Cannabis

1. https://stiffperson.org/?submissionGuid=8ecc3fc1-1e71-428a-a316-c1ef82443207

2. https://www.hopkinsmedicine.org/health/conditions-and-diseases/Stiff Person-syndrome-sps
3. https://www.ancient-origins.net/history-ancient-traditions/versatile-plant-what-were-many-uses-cannabis-ancient-egypt-007733
4. Russo, E. B., G. W. Guy, and P. J. Robson. 2007. Cannabis, pain, and sleep: Lessons from therapeutic clinical trials of Sativex, a cannabis-based medicine. Chemistry & Biodiversity 4(8):1729–1743.
5. IOM Institute of Medicine. 1999. Marijuana and medicine: Assessing the science base. Washington, DC: National Academy Press.
6. https://learn.taomc.org/cannabis-vs-marijuana-whats-the-difference/
7. https://www.ncbi.nlm.nih.gov/pmc/articles/PMC2626929/
8. https://onlinelibrary.wiley.com/doi/10.1111/j.1365-2710.2012.01365.x
9. Government of Canada. Information for health care professionals: cannabis and the cannabinoids. Secondary Information for healthcare professionals: cannabis and cannabinoids. 2018. www.canada.ca/content/dam/hc-sc/documents/services/drugs-medication/cannabis/information-medical-practitioners/information-health-care-professionals-cannabis-cannabinoids-eng.pdf.
10. Koppel, B. S., J. C. Brust, T. Fife, J. Bronstein, S. Youssof, G. Gronseth, and D. Gloss. 2014. Systematic review: Efficacy and safety of medical marijuana in selected neurologic disorders: Report of the Guideline Development Subcommittee of the American Academy of Neurology. Neurology 82(17):1556–1563.
11. https://www.sandiegouniontribune.com/sdut-calif-research-shows-pot-can-ease-muscle-spasms-2010feb17-story.html
12. https://pubmed.ncbi.nlm.nih.gov/23892791/
13. https://pubmed.ncbi.nlm.nih.gov/12137404/
14. https://www.ncbi.nlm.nih.gov/pmc/articles/PMC5764009/
15. https://pubmed.ncbi.nlm.nih.gov/29766748/

16. Patti F, Chisari C, D'Amico E, et al. Long-term effectiveness of 9-⊠-tetrahydrocannabinol: cannabidiol oromucosal spray in clinical practice: results from an 18-month multicenter Italian study. Poster presented at: 2019 American Academy of Neurology Annual Meeting; May 9, 2019; Philadelphia, PA.
17. Cannabis Information and Support. Weeding out the differences between THC vs. CBD.n.d.
18. *(McPartland, J. M. (2018). Cannabis Systematics at the Levels of Family, Genus, and Species. Cannabis and Cannabinoid Research, 3(1), 203-212. https://doi.org/10.1089/can.2018.0039 (https://www.rollingstone.com/culture/culture-features/andrew-huberman-cannabis-misinformation-slammed-by-experts-1235016613/)* Dosing
19. (https://www.nbcnews.com/politics/politics-news/reschedule-marijuana-drug-joe-biden-justice-department-rcna152603
20. https://www.forbes.com/sites/petersuciu/2020/02/07/cannabis-misinformation-spreading-on-social-media/)
21. (https://www.ama-assn.org/delivering-care/health-equity/how-legacy-medical-racism-shapes-us-health-care-today)
22. (https://www.drugs.com/drug-interactions/cannabis-index.html)

Chapter 4: Coping With the Pain, Stiffness, and Spasms of Stiff Person Syndrome

1. https://www.ncbi.nlm.nih.gov/pmc/articles/PMC3010965/
2. John Templeton Foundation by the Greater Good Science Center at UC Berkeley May 2018 The Science of Gratitude p. 4
3. www.iasp-pain.org/terminology
4. Gatchel et al., 2007
5. https://www.hss.edu/conditions_emotional-impact-pain experience.asp
6. https://psychcentral.com/health/types-of-endorphins
7. https://www.sciencedaily.com/releases/2020/10/201001133227.htm
8. https://pubmed.ncbi.nlm.nih.gov/23724462/

9. https://www.ncbi.nlm.nih.gov/pmc/articles/PMC5693231/
10. http://absentofi.org/2021/09/thich-nhat-hanh-you-embrace-your-pain-tenderly/
11. https://www.apa.org/topics/mindfulness/meditation
12. https://www.ncbi.nlm.nih.gov/books/NBK573078/#_NBK573078_ai__
13. https://rarediseases.org
14. https://www.ninds.nih.gov/about-ninds/who-we-are/ninds-mission
15. https://stiffperson.org
16. https://www.nychealthandhospitals.org/services/plant-based-lifestyle-medicine-program/
17. https://www.jumdjournal.net/article/view/2892

Chapter 4: LEARNING AND DISCUSSION

How To Cultivate Emotional Wellness

1. S., Crute (1997). Health and Healing for African Americans: Straight Talk and Tips from More Than 150 Black Doctors on Our Top Health Concerns (1st ed., pp. 424-425). Rodale Press.)
2. Williamson, L. (2022, January 3). The link between structural racism, high blood pressure, and Black People's Health. www.heart.org. https://www.heart.org/en/news/2021/04/15/the-link-between-structural-racism-high-blood-pressure-and-black-peoples-health) (Dixon, B. M. (1995). Good health for African Americans. Three Rivers Press.)
3. (C. C., Bell (2004). The Sanity of Survival Reflections on Community Mental Health and Wellness (1st ed., pp. 248-249). Third World Press.).
4. (Edwards MK, Loprinzi PD. Experimental effects of brief, single bouts of walking and meditation on mood profile in young adults. Health Promot Perspect. 2018 jul 7;8(3):171-178. doi: 10.15171/hpp.2018.23. PMID: 30087839; PMCID: PMC6064756)

   (del Pozo Cruz B, Ahmadi MN, Lee I, Stamatakis E. Prospective Associations of Daily Step Counts and Intensity With Cancer and Cardiovascular Disease Incidence and Mortality and All-Cause Mortality. JAMA Intern Med. 2022;182(11):1139–1148. doi:10.1001/jamainternmed.2022.4000).

5. Singh B, Olds T, Curtis R, Dumuid D, Virgara R, Watson A, Szeto K, O'Connor E, Ferguson T, Eglitis E, Miatke A, Simpson CE, Maher C. Effectiveness of physical activity interventions for improving depression, anxiety, and distress: an overview of systematic reviews. Br J Sports Med. 2023 Sep;57(18):1203-1209. doi: 10.1136/bjsports-2022-106195. Epub 2023 Feb 16. PMID: 36796860; PMCID: PMC10579187.) See (Jackson, Erica M. Ph.D., FACSM. STRESS RELIEF: The Role of Exercise in Stress Management. ACSM's Health & Fitness Journal 17(3):p 14-19, May/June 2013. | DOI: 10.1249/FIT.0b013e31828cb1c9)
6. Ellapen TJ, Hammill HV, Swanepoel M, Strydom GL. The health benefits and constraints of exercise therapy for wheelchair users: A clinical commentary. Afr J Disabil. 2017 Sep 8;6:337. Doi: 10.4102/ajod.v6i0.337. PMID: 28936414; PMCID: PMC5594262.)
7. Migala, J. (2024, July 18). Why are healthy eating habits important? EverydayHealth.com. https://www.everydayhealth.com/diet-nutrition/importance-healthy-eating-habits/) See (How dietary factors influence disease risk. (2017, March 21). National Institutes of Health (NIH). https://www.nih.gov/news-events/nih-research-matters/how-dietary-factors-influence-disease-risk
8. (Eating more ultra-processed foods tied to cognitive decline, stroke, according to study. (2024, May 24). ScienceDaily. https://www.sciencedaily.com/releases/2024/05/240522225300.htm)
9. Campbell, T. C., & Campbell, T. M. (2006). The China Study: The Most Comprehensive Study of Nutrition Ever Conducted and the Startling Implications for Diet, Weight Loss, and Long-term Health. BenBella Books.)
10. (Radavelli-Bagatini S, Blekkenhorst LC, Sim M, et al. Fruit and vegetable intake is inversely associated with perceived stress across the adult lifespan. Clinical Nutrition. 2021;40(5):2860-2867).
11. Puff, R. (2013, July 7). An Overview of Meditation: Its Origins and Traditions. Psychology Today. Retrieved July 26, 2024, from

https://www.psychologytoday.com/intl/blog/meditation-modern-life/201307/overview-meditation-its-origins-and-traditions) inversely associated with perceived stress across the adult lifespan. Clinical Nutrition. 2021;40(5):2860-2867).

12. Goyal M, Singh S, Sibinga EM, Gould NF, Rowland-Seymour A, Sharma R, Berger Z, Sleicher D, Maron DD, Shihab HM, Ranasinghe PD, Linn S, Saha S, Bass EB, Haythornthwaite JA. Meditation programs for psychological stress and well-being: a systematic review and meta-analysis. JAMA Intern Med. 2014 Mar;174(3):357-68. Doi: 10.1001/jamainternmed.2013.13018. PMID: 24395196; PMCID: PMC4142584.

    See (Jain FA, Walsh RN, Eisendrath SJ, Christensen S, Rael Cahn B. Critical analysis of the efficacy of meditation therapies for acute and subacute phase treatment of depressive disorders: a systematic review. Psychosomatics. 2015 Mar-Apr;56(2):140-52. doi: 10.1016/j.psym.2014.10.007. Epub 2014 Oct 22. PMID: 25591492; PMCID: PMC4383597.)

    See (Kiken LG, Shook NJ. Does mindfulness attenuate thoughts emphasizing negativity, but not positivity? J Res Pers. 2014 Dec 1;53:22-30. doi: 10.1016/j.jrp.2014.08.002. PMID: 25284906; PMCID: PMC4178287.)

    See (Kasala ER, Bodduluru LN, Maneti Y, Thipparaboina R. Effect of meditation on neurophysiological changes in stress-mediated depression. Complement Ther Clin Pract. 2014 Feb;20(1):74-80. doi: 10.1016/j.ctcp.2013.10.001. Epub 2013 Oct 18. PMID: 24439650.)

13. Goyal M, Singh S, Sibinga EM, Gould NF, Rowland-Seymour A, Sharma R, Berger Z, Sleicher D, Maron DD, Shihab HM, Ranasinghe PD, Linn S, Saha S, Bass EB, Haythornthwaite JA. Meditation programs for psychological stress and well-being: a systematic review and meta-analysis. JAMA Intern Med. 2014 Mar;174(3):357-68. Doi: 10.1001/jamainternmed.2013.13018. PMID: 24395196; PMCID: PMC4142584.

    See Rosenkranz, M. A., Davidson, R. J., Maccoon, D. G., Sheridan, J. F., Kalin, N. H., & Lutz, A. (2013). A comparison of mindfulness-based stress reduction and an active control in modulation of neurogenic inflammation. Brain, Behavior, and Immunity, 27, 174–184. https://doi.org/10.1016/j.bbi.2012.10.013)

See Cearley, S. M., Immaneni, S., & Shankar, P. (2017). Irritable Bowel Syndrome: The effect of FODMAPs and meditation on pain management. European Journal of Integrative Medicine, 12, 117–121. https://doi.org/10.1016/j.eujim.2017.05.003)

See Hilton L, Maher AR, Colaiaco B, Apaydin E, Sorbero ME, Booth M, Shanman RM, Hempel S. Meditation for posttraumatic stress: Systematic review and meta-analysis. Psychol Trauma. 2017 Jul;9(4):453-460. doi: 10.1037/tra0000180. Epub 2016 Aug 18. PMID: 27537781.)

See Aman MM, Jason Yong R, Kaye AD, Urman RD. Evidence-Based Non-Pharmacological Therapies for Fibromyalgia. Curr Pain Headache Rep. 2018 Apr 4;22(5):33. doi: 10.1007/s11916-018-0688-2. PMID: 29619620.)

See Mindfulness meditation: A research-proven way to reduce stress. (2019, October 30). https://www.apa.org. https://www.apa.org/topics/mindfulness/meditation)

See (MacDonald, A. (2010, November 11). Using the relaxation response to reduce stress. Harvard Health. https://www.health.harvard.edu/blog/using-the-relaxation-response-to-reduce-stress-20101110780#app)

14. Bai Z, Chang J, Chen C, Li P, Yang K, Chi I. Investigating the effect of transcendental meditation on blood pressure: a systematic review and meta-analysis. J Hum Hypertens. 2015 Nov;29(11):653-62. Doi: 10.1038/jhh.2015.6. Epub 2015 Feb 12. PMID: 25673114.

    See Olex S, Newberg A, Figueredo VM. Meditation: should a cardiologist care? Int J Cardiol. 2013 Oct 3;168(3):1805-10. doi: 10.1016/j.ijcard.2013.06.086. Epub 2013 Jul 24. PMID: 23890919.)

    See Harvard Health. (2023, July 18). Meditation and a relaxation technique to lower blood pressure. https://www.health.harvard.edu/heart-health/meditation-and-a-relaxation-technique-to-lower-blood-pressure)

15. Khalsa, D. S. (2015). Stress, meditation, and Alzheimer's Disease Prevention: Where the evidence stands. Journal of Alzheimer's Disease, 48(1), 1–12. https://doi.org/10.3233/jad-142766

See Gard T, Hölzel BK, Lazar SW. The potential effects of meditation on age-related cognitive decline: a systematic review. Ann N Y Acad Sci. 2014 Jan;1307:89-103. doi: 10.1111/nyas.12348. PMID: 24571182; PMCID: PMC4024457.

See Hurley RV, Patterson TG, Cooley SJ. Meditation-based interventions for family caregivers of people with dementia: a review of the empirical literature. Aging Ment Health. 2014;18(3):281-8. doi: 10.1080/13607863.2013.837145. Epub 2013 Oct 6. PMID: 24093954.

See Norris CJ, Creem D, Hendler R, Kober H. Brief Mindfulness Meditation Improves Attention in Novices: Evidence From ERPs and Moderation by Neuroticism. Front Hum Neurosci. 2018 Aug 6;12:315. doi: 10.3389/fnhum.2018.00315. Erratum in: Front Hum Neurosci. 2018 Sep 05;12:342. doi: 10.3389/fnhum.2018.00342. PMID: 30127731; PMCID: PMC6088366.

See Tsai SY, Jaiswal S, Chang CF, Liang WK, Muggleton NG, Juan CH. Meditation Effects on the Control of Involuntary Contingent Reorienting Revealed With Electroencephalographic and Behavioral Evidence. Front Integr Neurosci. 2018 May 15;12:17. doi: 10.3389/fnint.2018.00017. PMID: 29867385; PMCID: PMC5962705.

See Sood A, Jones DT. On mind wandering, attention, brain networks, and meditation. Explore (NY). 2013 May-Jun;9(3):136-41. doi: 10.1016/j.explore.2013.02.005. PMID: 23643368.

See Basso JC, McHale A, Ende V, Oberlin DJ, Suzuki WA. Brief, daily meditation enhances attention, memory, mood, and emotional regulation in non-experienced meditators. Behav Brain Res. 2019 Jan 1;356:208-220. doi: 10.1016/j.bbr.2018.08.023. Epub 2018 Aug 25. PMID: 30153464.

16. Black DS, Slavich GM. Mindfulness meditation and the immune system: a systematic review of randomized controlled trials. Ann

N Y Acad Sci. 2016 Jun;1373(1):13-24. doi: 10.1111/nyas.12998. Epub 2016 Jan 21. PMID: 26799456; PMCID: PMC4940234.

See Chandran, V., Bermúdez, M., Koka, M., Chandran, B., Pawale, D., Vishnubhotla, R., Alankar, S., Maturi, R., Subramaniam, B., & Sadhasivam, S. (2021). Large-scale genomic study reveals robust activation of the immune system following advanced Inner Engineering meditation retreat. Proceedings of the National Academy of Sciences, 118(51), e2110455118. https://doi.org/10.1073/pnas.2110455118)

See Davidson RJ, Kabat-Zinn J, Schumacher J, Rosenkranz M, Muller D, Santorelli SF, Urbanowski F, Harrington A, Bonus K, Sheridan JF. Alterations in brain and immune function produced by mindfulness meditation. Psychosom Med. 2003 Jul-Aug;65(4):564-70. doi: 10.1097/01.psy.0000077505.67574.e3. PMID: 12883106.)

17. Hilton L, Hempel S, Ewing BA, Apaydin E, Xenakis L, Newberry S, Colaiaco B, Maher AR, Shanman RM, Sorbero ME, Maglione MA. Mindfulness Meditation for Chronic Pain: Systematic Review and Meta-analysis. Ann Behav Med. 2017 Apr;51(2):199-213. doi: 10.1007/s12160-016-9844-2. PMID: 27658913; PMCID: PMC5368208.

    See Goyal M, Singh S, Sibinga EM, Gould NF, Rowland-Seymour A, Sharma R, Berger Z, Sleicher D, Maron DD, Shihab HM, Ranasinghe PD, Linn S, Saha S, Bass EB, Haythornthwaite JA. Meditation programs for psychological stress and well-being: a systematic review and meta-analysis. JAMA Intern Med. 2014 Mar;174(3):357-68. doi: 10.1001/jamainternmed.2013.13018. PMID: 24395196; PMCID: PMC4142584.)

18. Orme-Johnson DW, Barnes VA. Effects of the transcendental meditation technique on trait anxiety: a meta-analysis of randomized controlled trials. J Altern Complement Med. 2014 May;20(5):330-41. doi: 10.1089/acm.2013.0204. Epub 2013 Oct 9. PMID: 24107199.

    See Hoge EA, Bui E, Marques L, Metcalf CA, Morris LK, Robinaugh DJ, Worthington JJ, Pollack MH, Simon NM.

Randomized controlled trial of mindfulness meditation for generalized anxiety disorder: effects on anxiety and stress reactivity. J Clin Psychiatry. 2013 Aug;74(8):786-92. doi: 10.4088/JCP.12m08083. PMID: 23541163; PMCID: PMC3772979.

See Rod K. Observing the Effects of Mindfulness-Based Meditation on Anxiety and Depression in Chronic Pain Patients. Psychiatr Danub. 2015 Sep;27 Suppl 1:S209-11. PMID: 26417764.

See Hofmann SG, Gómez AF. Mindfulness-Based Interventions for Anxiety and Depression. Psychiatr Clin North Am. 2017 Dec;40(4):739-749. doi: 10.1016/j.psc.2017.08.008. Epub 2017 Sep 18. PMID: 29080597; PMCID: PMC5679245.

See Bostock S, Crosswell AD, Prather AA, Steptoe A. Mindfulness on-the-go: Effects of a mindfulness meditation app on work stress and well-being. J Occup Health Psychol. 2019 Feb;24(1):127-138. doi: 10.1037/ocp0000118. Epub 2018 May 3. PMID: 29723001; PMCID: PMC6215525.)

19. Jason C. Ong, Rachel Manber, Zindel Segal, Yinglin Xia, Shauna Shapiro, James K. Wyatt, A Randomized Controlled Trial of Mindfulness Meditation for Chronic Insomnia, Sleep, Volume 37, Issue 9, 1 September 2014, Pages 1553–1563, https://doi.org/10.5665/sleep.4010

20. Boelens, P. A., Reeves, R. R., Replogle, W. H., & Koenig, H. G. (2012). The Effect of Prayer on Depression and Anxiety: Maintenance of Positive Influence One Year after Prayer Intervention. International Journal of Psychiatry in Medicine, 43(1), 85–98. https://doi.org/10.2190/pm.43.1.f

    See Moreira-Almeida, A., Sharma, A., Van Rensburg, B. J., Verhagen, P. J., & Cook, C. C. (2016). WPA Position Statement on Spirituality and Religion in Psychiatry. World Psychiatry, 15(1), 87–88. https://doi.org/10.1002/wps.20304)

    See Nadi, M., & Ghahremani, N. (2014). The relationship between dimensions of religiosity/spirituality with mental health and hope for the future between staff of public hospitals in Shiraz. Journal of Education and Health Promotion, 3(1), 20. https://doi.org/10.4103/2277-9531.127600

See Ottaviani, A. C., Souza, É. N., De Camargo Drago, N., De Mendiondo, M. S. Z., Pavarini, S. C. I., & De Souza Orlandi, F. (2014). Hope and spirituality among patients with chronic kidney disease undergoing hemodialysis: a correlational study. Revista Latino-americana De Enfermagem, 22(2), 248–254. https://doi.org/10.1590/0104-1169.3323.2409)

21. Amen, D. G., MD. (2010). Change your brain, change your body: Use Your Brain to Get and Keep the Body You Have Always Wanted. Harmony.
22. Goh, C. (2024, July 19). Your Breath is Your Brain's Remote Control. Mindful. https://www.mindful.org/breath-brains-remote-control/

    See (Zelano, C., Jiang, H., Zhou, G., Arora, N., Schuele, S., Rosenow, J., & Gottfried, J. A. (2016). Nasal respiration entrains human limbic oscillations and modulates cognitive function. Journal of Neuroscience, 36(49), 12448–12467. https://doi.org/10.1523/jneurosci.2586-16.2016)

Chapter 5: Stiff Person Syndrome and Sexual Health

1. Glasier A, Gulmezogfu AM, Schmid GP, Garcia Moreno C, Van Look PFA. Sexual and reproductive health: a matter of life and death. Lancet. 2006;368 (9547):1595-607. Also, Lee DM, Nazroo J, O'Connor DB, Blake M, Pendleton N. Sexual health and well-being among older men and women in England: findings from the English longitudinal study of aging. Arch Sex Behav. 2016;45(1):133–44
2. https://www.ncbi.nlm.nih.gov/pmc/articles/PMC5963213/; https://pubmed.ncbi.nlm.nih.gov/31494914/; https://pubmed.ncbi.nlm.nih.gov/31432361/; https://www.sciencedirect.com/science/article/abs/pii/S1743609515334457
3. https://www.ncbi.nlm.nih.gov/pmc/articles/PMC7489086/
4. https://tallirosenbaum.com/2016/12/22/in-sickness-and-in-health-intimacy-and-chronic-illness/
5. https://cardiacrehab.ucsf.edu/sexual-activity-and-your-heart
6. World Health Organization, 1995

7. https://hhma.org/healthadvisor/aha-sexinmen-crs/
8. https://nationalhealthcouncil.org/wp-content/uploads/2019/12/AboutChronicDisease.pdf
9. https://www.cambridge.org/core/journals/advances-in-psychiatric-treatment/article/sexual-dysfunction-classification-and-assessment/3227B0096B40B7445E851B181F03109E
10. Schover LR. Sexual problems in chronic illness. In: Leiblum SR, Rosen RC, eds. Principles and practice of sex therapy. 3d ed. New York: Guilford, 2000: 398–422); Wandell PE, Brorsson B. Assessing sexual functioning in patients with chronic disorders by using a generic health-related quality of life questionnaire. Qual Life Res. 2000;9:1081-92; https://www.aafp.org/pubs/afp/issues/2003/0115/p347.html#afp20030115p347-b13
11. https://www.sciencedirect.com/science/article/abs/pii/S0735675796901588?via%3Dihub
12. https://my.clevelandclinic.org/health/diseases/9121-sexual-dysfunction
13. Yeniel A, Petri E. Pregnancy, childbirth, and sexual function: Perceptions and facts. Int Urogynecol J 2014; 25: 5–14; https://www.contemporaryobgyn.net/view/how-prevalent-are-sexual-problems-among-middle-aged-canadians
14. https://www.uhhospitals.org/blog/articles/2021/02/women-dont-have-to-tolerate-sexual-dysfunction#:~:text=One%20in%2010%20women%20have,Often%2C%20these%20problems%20overlap.
15. https://www.ncbi.nlm.nih.gov/pmc/articles/PMC8261092/
16. https://www.sciencedirect.com/science/article/pii/S0753332218353289
17. https://www.nm.org/conditions-and-care-areas/urology/sexual-dysfunction.
18. Based on data reviewed as part of Macmillan Cancer Support (2013) Throwing light on the consequences of cancer and its treatment: Department of Health. 2012. Quality of Life of Cancer Survivors

in England. Report on a pilot survey using Patient Reported Outcome Measures (PROMS) and UK cancer prevalence data.

19. https://journals.plos.org/plosone/article?id=10.1371/journal.pone.0282618; Lee DM, Nazroo J, O'Connor DB, Blake M, Pendleton N. Sexual health and well-being among older men and women in England: findings from the English longitudinal study of aging. Arch Sex Behav. 2016;45(1):133–44. pmid:25624001; Graham CA, Štulhofer A, Lange T, Hald GM, Carvalheira AA, Enzlin P, et al. Prevalence and predictors of sexual difficulties and associated distress among partnered, sexually active older women in Norway, Denmark, Belgium, and Portugal. Quinn-Nilas C, Milhausen RR, McKay A, Holzapfel S. Prevalence and predictors of sexual problems among midlife Canadian adults: results from a national survey. J Sex Med. 2018;15(6):873-9.pmid:29753802
20. https://blackdoctor.org/stress-relieving-sex-positions/?_kx=1WhkTyi9yLQh6w7E32qGdBjqAFWd4HSQbdMSzRmBUg4%3D.NqNqSV
21. http://authors.simonandschuster.com/Zane/269527
22. Dr. Thomas Moore, "Soul Mates," *Psychology Today*, (Mar/Apr 1994), pp. 28, 29.
23. https://www.bodyandsoul.comau/sex-relationships/sex/the-worlds-first-hands-free-sex-toyhas-been-designed-for-those-with-disabilities/news-story/1d6bf50e80a42c85coa753oc28253882
24. https://health.cornell.edu/sites/health/files/pdf-library/sensate-focus.pdf
25. https://my.clevelandclinic.org/health/diseases/9123-sexual-dysfunction-in-females; https://www.aafp.org/pubs/afp/issues/2003/0115/p347.html#afp20030115p347-b7); www.zestraforwomen.com; https://www.health.harvard.edu/staying-healthy/11-ways-to-help-yourself-to-a-better-sex-life
26. https://www.mayoclinic.org/diseases-conditions/erectile-dysfunction/diagnosis-treatment/drc-20355782

27. https://www.bcm.edu/research/research-centers/center-for-research-on-women-with-disabilities/a-to-z-directory/sexual-health/sex-surrogates;https://www.ncbi.nlm.nih.gov/pmc/articles/PMC10212222/; (https://www.essence.com/lifestyle/sex-doulas/

28. (Joshi AM, Arkiath Veettil R, Deshpande S. Role of Yoga in the Management of Premature Ejaculation. World J Mens Health. 2020 Oct;38(4):495-505. doi: 10.5534/wjmh.190062. Epub 2019 Sep 3. PMID: 31496152; PMCID: PMC7502310.) (Morales-Brown, L. (2024, August 6). Everything you need to know about tantric sex. https://www.medicalnewstoday.com/articles/what-is-tantric-sex)

29. https://www.jocelynleestudio.com/sovereign

30. (Dixon, P. (2007). African American Relationships, Marriages, and Families: An Introduction. New York: Routledge.)

31. (Minirth, F. B., PhD, & Newman, B. (1994). Passages of Marriages: Five Growth Stages That Will Take Your Marriage to Greater Intimacy. Nelsonword Publishing Group.)

32. (Marshall, T. C. (2008). Cultural differences in intimacy: The influence of gender-role ideology and individualism-collectivism. Journal of Social and Personal Relationships, 25, 143–169. doi: 10.1177/0265407507086810) (Rokach, A. (2023). Love Culturally: How Does Culture Affect Intimacy, Commitment & Love. The Journal of Psychology, 158(1), 84–114. https://doi.org/10.1080/00223980.2023.2244129)

33. (Harvard Health. (2023a, June 13). Oxytocin: The love hormone. https://www.health.harvard.edu/mind-and-mood/oxytocin-the-love-hormone)

34. (Karandashev, V. (2015). A Cultural Perspective on Romantic Love. Online Readings in Psychology and Culture, 5(4). https://doi.org/10.9707/2307-0919.1135)

Chapter 6: On Laughter

1. Cousins, Norman, Anatomy of an illness as perceived by the patient: reflections on healing and regeneration, intro. by René Dubos, New York: Norton, 1979. ISBN 0-393-01252-2.

2. http://berniesiegelmd.com/2021/08/tears-of-joy/
3. https://www.henryford.com/blog/2019/03/how-laughter-benefits-heart-health
4. https://www.health.harvard.edu/mind-and-mood/feel-good-hormones-how-they-affect-your-mind-mood-and-body
5. https://pubmed.ncbi.nlm.nih.gov/16319105/
6. https://pubmed.ncbi.nlm.nih.gov/12652882/
7. https://diabetesjournals.org/care/article/26/5/1651/24552/Laughter-Lowered-the-Increase-in-Postprandial
8. https://www.psychologytoday.com/us/blog/sleeping-angels/201205/why-laughing-in-the-evening-helps-you-sleep-better-night
9. https://pubmed.ncbi.nlm.nih.gov/35782290/
10. https://www.wiesenthal.com/about/about-simon-wiesenthal/
11. https://www.scientificamerican.com/article/laugh-lots-live-longer/
12. Kim SH, Kook JR, Kwon M, Son MH, Ahn SD, Kim YH. The effects of laughter therapy on mood state and self-esteem in cancer patients undergoing radiation therapy: a randomized controlled trial. J Altern Complement Med. 2015;21(4):217-22).
13. Kimata H. Effect of viewing a humorous vs. nonhumorous film on bronchial responsiveness in patients with bronchial asthma. Physiol Behav. 2004;81(4):681-684.
14. Brutsche MH, Grossman P, Muller RE, et al. Impact of laughter on air trapping in severe chronic obstructive lung disease. Int J Chron Obstruct Pulmon Dis. 2008;3(1):185-192.
15. https://www.semanticscholar.org/paper/Humors-Effect-on-Short-term-Memory-in-Healthy-and-Bains-Berk/5938d6d07b2d9ad7e2394227611233c899d92e50.
16. Bega D, Palmentera P, Wagner A, et al. Laughter is the best medicine: The Second City((R)) improvisation as an intervention for Parkinson's disease. Parkinsonism Relat Disord. 2017;34:62-65.
17. https://europepmc.org/article/MED/25266473

18. https://medium.com/joincurio/sometimes-its-better-to-laugh-with-a-friend-rather-than-laughing-alone-102e387b9d09.
19. https://www.laughteronlineuniversity.com/social-benefits-laughter/
20. https://www.bluezones.com/2011/10/laugh-therapy-new-secret-to-longevity/.
21. https://www.ppccfl.com/blog/threat-or-challenge.
22. Skinner N, Brewer N. The Dynamics of Threat and Challenge Appraisals Prior to Stressful Achievement Events. Journal of Personality and Social Psychology.
23. https://www.stlfertility.com/laughter-is-contagious-like-a-virus/
24. (Heasman, C. (2023, February 2). Foods that look amazing but taste terrible. Mashed. https://www.mashed.com/64366/foods-look-amazing-actually-taste-terrible/)
25. (Kataria, M. (n.d.). Laughter Yoga International: Promoting health, happiness, and peace through laughter. Laughter Yoga International. https://www.laughteryoga.org/)
26. (Today's Comics Online | Read comic strips at GoComics. (n.d.). https://www.gocomics.com/)
27. (Saturday Night Live - NBC.com. (n.d.). NBC. https://www.nbc.com/saturday-night-live)

Chapter 7: Final Thoughts

1. Hunter, K. (February 22, 2023). Dr. Daniel Black: After the Show with Tim in Dallas. [Karen Hunter Show]. https://thehub.news/dr-daniel-black-after-the-show-with-tim-in-dallas/

ACKNOWLEDGMENTS

This book is a testament to my transformation from doctor to patient, and I cannot express enough gratitude for those who have helped me along the way. My wife, Denise, deserves special thanks for her encouragement and understanding as I worked long hours finishing this book. She somehow knew when to ask about my progress and when it was better to talk about something else. I am forever grateful for her love and support. To my daughters, Dominique Scott, Alexis Hickman, and Arianne Benford: thank you all for listening to me talk about the book and for giving me your unwavering support. Ronald Allen, Dr. Rachel Anderson, Tanya Davis, Ruth Fornasiere, Pamela Gee Hall, Stephen Knox, Dana Noel, Joseph Williams, and Louis Holland Jr. read every word of the manuscript—some more than once—and offered invaluable feedback on my thoughts and interpretations. An extra-special recognition goes out to sociologist Dr. Henry Allen and editor Walter Leavy for their skillful and insightful commentary; I truly appreciate their contributions that are etched within the book's pages. You are both exceptional writers and authors.

I express my gratitude to the people who have educated me; my patients and students for what I have learned from them (some stories I tell in this book), and my mentors and peers for teaching me the principles of clinical psychology.

I owe a tremendous appreciation to my editor, Sarah Bass, who worked tirelessly to bring this book project to fruition. Without her leadership, this endeavor would have been doomed to failure. She listened patiently to my concerns and gave me sage advice. Draft after draft of the manuscript was read with scrupulous attention given to the sequencing, organization, grammar, and punctuation. Her talents are extraordinary, and her counsel was always spot on.

Finally, I want to sincerely thank Patrice Samara, Marva Allen, and the entire team at my publisher, Wordeee, for paving the way for the aspiration to come true. Your kind words, understanding of the vision, and expertise in enhancing the book's clarity and conformation to style without compromising its voice were invaluable. Patrice, you are a masterful teacher. Thank you for being accessible and encouraging me to see this journey to the end. Marva, your keen eye, and sharp attention to the manuscript's details were irreplaceable.

ABOUT THE AUTHOR

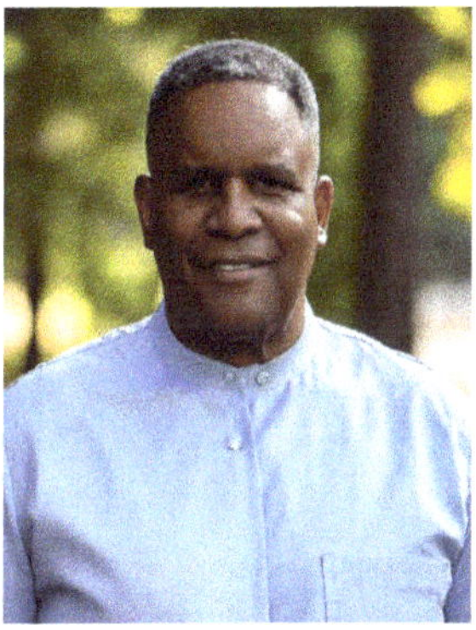

Tracy Scott, Psy.D., is a celebrated lecturer, scholar, and teacher who has been lauded internationally throughout many communities for his contributions to helping those most in need benefit from a holistic approach to human development and mental and spiritual health.

Dr. Scott earned his doctorate in clinical psychology from the Alfred Adler Institute of Chicago (now Adler University). He completed his internship in clinical psychology at the Minirth-Meier Clinic in Wheaton, IL, and also completed a two-year postdoctoral fellowship in clinical neuropsychology at Schwab Rehabilitation Hospital in Chicago, Illinois.

With additional advanced education and training in psychopharmacology and clinical spiritual counseling, Dr. Scott has written several articles on a variety of topics and hosted various radio programs. He has created and hosted national radio programs such as Wisdom for Joyous Living, Ask the Doctors, and Life Perspectives. For several years, he was a featured weekly guest on WGLB AM 1560, Milwaukee, WI; KAVH 101.5 FM, Eudora, AK and Internet Radio.

Throughout his professional career, he has delivered presentations and facilitated discussions across the country and internationally on a range of significant topics, including *"Where the Mind Goes, Behavior Follows," "Phantom Limb Syndrome," "Strokes and Hypertension," "Cancer and African Americans," "Treatment of Hyperglycemia and Managing Weight Gain with the Use of Atypical Medications," "Managing Stress," "Sexual Dysfunction," "Spinal Cord Injury," "Psychological Aspects of Traumatic Brain Injury," "Overcoming Anxiety and Depression," "Post Traumatic Stress Disorder the Result of Genocide,"* and *"Understanding and Managing Unwanted Thoughts."* His work encompasses various aspects of mental, biopsychosocial, and spiritual health issues, reflecting a deep commitment to enhancing understanding and awareness in these critical areas.

Additionally, as an active member of his community, he has published and provided resources on:

- *Tips for Managing Stress*
- *Domestic Violence: The Problem We Refuse to Face*
- *Growing Through Adversity & Plagues*
- *Strategies for a Successful Marriage*
- *Encouraging Hope for Substance Abusers and Their Families*
- *Coping with Chronic Illness with Faith and Prayer*
- *Life on a Roller Coaster: Managing Diabetes*
- *Suicide: A Challenge to Ministry*
- *How to Prevent Yourself from Singing the Holiday Blues*

Dr. Scott is a retired Senior Lecturer at Loyola University Chicago. He resides in southwest Florida with his supportive and creative wife, Denise.

Diagnosed with Stiff Person Syndrome (SPS) in 2017, he has dedicated his life to helping others living with SPS or other chronic illnesses. He enjoys practicing tai chi, biking, maintaining a whole-food, plant-based lifestyle, and listening to jazz.

www.ingramcontent.com/pod-product-compliance
Lightning Source LLC
Chambersburg PA
CBHW041302210926
51847CB00010B/112
9781959811602